AF327241

Nursing Home Staff Development

Nora S. Ernst is on the faculty at the University of Texas Health Science Center at Dallas, with a joint appointment in Allied Health Education and Gerontology. She holds a Ph.D. in educational research and evaluation and has worked in educational gerontology for the past five years. Her research has included a survey of Texas training coordinators, which was supported by a multi-year grant. As a result of this research, continuing education and college programs have been developed. Her teaching includes the areas of evaluation, needs assessment, and the development of training programs. She is the author/editor of numerous teaching materials in gerontology for allied health students, and is researching the development of gerontology education for allied health professionals.

Helen L. West holds a Ph.D. in education and gerontology and an M.A. in psychology. She is a licensed nursing home administrator in Texas and, since 1975, has been assistant professor in the Gerontology Services Administration Program at the University of Texas Health Science Center at Dallas. Her teaching responsibilities involve various aspects of long-term care administration, preparing students to become nursing home administrators. Prior to her university affiliation, Dr. West was a staff psychologist for a nursing home which became a model training facility for the Department of Health and Human Services, Region VI. During the time the nursing home functioned as a training facility, Dr. West was the training program director.

Dr. West's research interests center on the theme of improving the quality of life for older people in general, and especially for those who are institutionalized. As an expansion of this interest, Dr. West cofounded a life enrichment program for older adults.

Nursing Home Staff Development

A Guide for Inservice Programs

Nora S. Ernst, Ph.D.
Helen L. West, Ph.D.

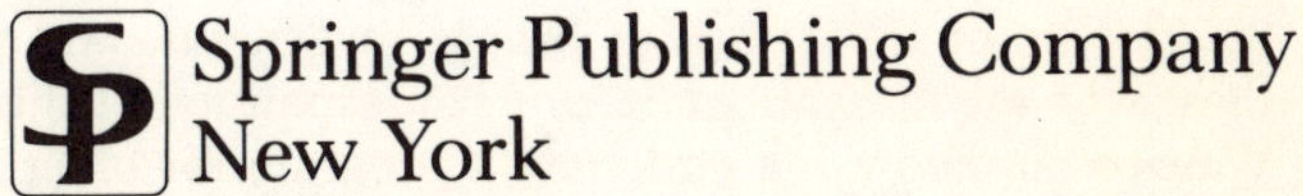

Springer Publishing Company
New York

Copyright © 1983 by Springer Publishing Company, Inc.

All rights reserved

No part of this publication may be reproduced, stored in a retrieval system, or transmitted in any form or by any means, electronic, mechanical, photocopying, recording, or otherwise, without the prior permission of Springer Publishing Company, Inc.

Springer Publishing Company, Inc.
200 Park Avenue South
New York, New York 10003

83 84 85 86 87 / 10 9 8 7 6 5 4 3 2 1

Library of Congress Cataloging in Publication Data

Ernst, Nora S.
   Nursing home staff development.

   Includes bibliographies and index.
   1. Nursing homes—Employees—In-service training.
I. West, Helen L.   II. Title.   [DNLM: 1. Inservice
training.   2. Nursing homes—Organization.   WX 159 E65n]
RA999.I5E76   1983   362.1'6'0683   82-10721
ISBN 0-8261-3860-8

Printed in the United States of America

Contents

Preface

Several years ago, the state of Texas passed legislation requiring that every nursing home in the state designate an inservice coordinator in order to be eligible for financial reimbursement. Since the legislation was passed, nursing homes have complied with the requirement, providing inservice for all employees. Specific topics were also required for all staff who were involved with the nursing home residents.

This book is designed to provide an overview of the educational components involved in inservice development, delivery, and evaluation. Inservice in the nursing home is discussed within the context of the home and its benefits to the home. The overall educational model of needs assessment, planning, delivery, and evaluation is used as the structural basis for a discussion of specific topics. Also included is the area of adult education as well as the often overlooked delivery methods of role play, case study, simulation, and outside resources. It is the authors' hope that this book will provide the framework for beneficial, ongoing inservice for nursing home personnel.

The authors wish to recognize the Research Coordinating Unit, Department of Occupational Education and Technology, Texas Education Agency. Without their support, the initial research and development of the materials that has resulted in *Nursing Home Staff Development* could not have been done.

Chapter 1

Inservice Coordination in the Nursing Home

An inservice director is a teacher-manager. Sometimes the director's role will be primarily that of a teacher, at other times primarily a manager and a coordinator. The role will vary from day to day, from department to department, and from nursing home to nursing home. The inservice director must be a flexible multi-talented person. No matter what the circumstances, basic knowledge of the various aspects of inservice is essential.

As a teacher the inservice director will be responsible for much of the actual teaching. Supervision of other teachers, organization of the technical aspects of teaching, and familiarization with subject content may also be expected. As a manager, learner outcomes and personal relations with learners and the nursing home's patients will be of importance. Other important aspects of the role of inservice director include awareness of professional and community developments within long-term care, the ability to effectively plan for both the present and the future, to employ and maintain top quality effort and efficiency. An inservice director cannot expect more of learners than of himself.* Leadership skills are of utmost importance. The ability to delegate work and authority quickly, effectively and inexpensively is vital. This will promote maximum efficiency. The director must know and understand how to select and develop manpower. The ability to coordinate all the operations of a particular work area so that all personnel work together effectively is essential. In order for this to happen, effective communication to all levels of personnel regarding inservice and procedures must be undertaken. A good knowledge of language will be of help. An inservice director must be able to get the most out of the available literature and be able to translate that material into a level that is appropriate and learnable for different learners.

Last, an inservice director must understand the organization, be knowledgeable of the policies of the particular institution as well as any relevant government regulations. Inservice must be part of, and supported by, administration and supervisory staff. The inservice director may be asked to motivate employees, work with administration, teach, learn, coordinate, and perform a myriad of additional tasks. A thorough understanding of people will make all of these tasks possible.

A Definition of Inservice

It has been said that inservice education in nursing homes is a systematic and continuing process of providing job-related learning experiences for all personnel responsible for direct and indirect care and services to patient/residents (United Hospital Fund of New York, 1972). When thus viewed the

---

*Throughout this book, the masculine pronoun has been used for convenience, with the understanding that it is meant to include women as well as men.

concept of inservice education seems to be something of a monolith, a task bigger than life that can never be fully understood or completed. But, as with all complex processes, thorough inservice education is within the grasp of any nursing home. The secret is that all aspects of the facility must be willing to work at it. In order to achieve this coordinated effort, the trainer must break this broad concept into specific, one-step-at-a-time objectives.

In the nursing home the ultimate goal of inservice education is to improve the quality of life for the residents. An inservice education program should focus on increasing the technical proficiency and social communication skills of the nursing home staff, as well as keeping the staff up to date on new techniques, equipment, and concepts of care. The program should be meticulously planned rather than haphazardly thrown together.

Inservice education can encompass the following four major areas:

1. *Orientation* to the home's specific objectives, organization, personnel policies, job descriptions, and to the physical plant in which care and services are provided to patient/residents. This includes ongoing orientation of all personnel to any changes in the nursing home.
2. *Skill Training* to develop competencies related to physical needs of patient/residents; for example, nursing care, food service, activities of daily living, safety, application of written procedures for care of persons with acute or chronic illnesses, including rehabilitative and restorative techniques.
3. *Continuing Education* to build additional competencies and to integrate interpersonal skills into all aspects of interaction with patient/residents, families, other visitors to the home, other personnel from various departments within the home, etc. Continuing education provides new

knowledge, understanding, and skills based on findings of research in the physical and behavioral sciences; for example, new techniques for serving physical, social, emotional, and spiritual needs of institutionalized aging persons with illnesses or disabilities.

4. *Leadership and Management Development* for selected personnel who show potential for learning and applying new methods of leadership and for those in management positions who show evidence of need for assistance in this area of on-the-job performance (United Hospital Fund of New York, 1972).

Orientation

Orientation gives employees basic information to help them to function efficiently and effectively within the nursing home. Each employee needs to know and understand organizational policies, procedures, structure, services, and benefits. The length and depth of orientation will vary among nursing homes depending on size, specialized services, number of employees, and the knowledge and skills of new employees.

Orientation is both a welcome and an introduction. It is the time during which the new employee is introduced to supervisers and colleagues. The orientation program should include an introduction to the home and the home's policies, procedures, personnel, and physical facilities and should instill in employees a positive attitude of belonging in the organization. It should also clarify the new employee's job description; provide instruction adequate to aid the employee to begin the job with confidence and security; introduce performance expectations both within departments and in the facility as a whole. In this way new employees are famliarized with their own department, its functions, its relationship with other departments, its supervisory staff, and with working colleagues.

To achieve this, it is extremely important that the department supervisor inform present employees of several things: that a new person has been hired; the rationale for hiring the new person; and the new employee's function within the department. This will set the stage and help create a positive work environment for the new employee.

There are other ways to ease the adjustment of a new employee. An inservice director can develop an employee orientation manual to be given to each new employee. This manual would list and explain personal policy, facility services, benefits and programs. An individual department information packet containing the organizational chart for the department, the new employee's job description, departmental procedures, regulations, and a listing of staff members with their titles can also be of help. New employees' names may be announced on departmental bulletin boards and in the facility newspaper. A department buddy system, in which established staff members serve as resource agents for new employees, can also be organized.

Before a staff member begins an inservice education program, however, he must be familiar with the facility, the routine, the regulations, and the people with whom he will work. Orientation, like inservice education, should never be haphazard. A thorough, well-rounded orientation program will eliminate countless problems for new employees.

Skill Training

Skill training ensures that all employees have basic work skills. Although some employees may come to the facility with previous experience and training, others may need skill training. The length and depth of skill training depends on the facility, the employee, and the inservice organization.

Skill training develops basic competencies for patient care

and should be regarded as a vital component of both new employee orientation and ongoing staff development. The ultimate goal of skill training should encompass all basic patient care skills needed in order to perform a job effectively and efficiently.

The basic steps in developing skill training are listed below. Each step is essential.

1. Determine needed skills. Ask the administrator, the supervisor, and the employee what skills are most needed. Check state and federal guidelines. Determine what the employee can and cannot do.
2. Observe current level of performance. Observe the employee as he performs an actual job. Ask the employee to demonstrate skills that have not been observed.
3. Teach and reevaluate. Wherever and whenever, demonstrate needed skills. Where there are deficiencies, provide ongoing training. Ask supervisors to demonstrate and check progress. Be a good role model.
4. Review monitors of performance. Incident reports, financial statements, supervisory reviews, patients' comments are all informative. Never be satisfied with skills. Constantly update, review, and develop skills.

Continuing Education

Continuing education helps employees to develop new skills and to increase job competency. It provides new knowledge and skills that enhance minimum job performance and encourage optimum job performance. It is an essential component of staff development and should be an ongoing, never ending activity of the facility.

Continuing education has four general goals. The first goal is to update new or changing facets of the facility, its policies, procedures, and personnel. Next, continuing education provides information on recent developments including new techniques and new medications within a given field of work. Developing employees' attitudes toward the facility, its employees, its patients, and the community is a third goal. Personal growth and development which help an employee reach full job potential is also a goal. To achieve these goals the inservice trainer should have an ongoing interesting program. Employees should want to attend and feel that training is relevant and rewarding. Ways in which an inservice director can foster this attitude are:

1. Be sure that the learning experience is both needed and relevant. Conduct a formal or informal needs assessment to determine specific knowledge and skill level needed by employers. Do not produce learning experiences that are above or below employee capabilities or job roles.
2. Gain administrative and supervisory support. When the management views inservice as vital, so do the employees.
3. Use the past knowledge and experiences of the employee whenever possible. When those experiences are not directly related to the present situation, try whenever possible to transfer attitudes and parallel skills.
4. Be sensitive and respectful of employees' time. Continuing education should start on time, have a prepared agenda, and should have stated, specific objectives.
5. Relate the learning content directly to the employee's job. This will help the employees to see the relevance and utilization of continuing education.

Continuing education should be presented through a variety of methods; these should aid employees in mastering the learning objectives. Individual meetings, class attendance, peer tutoring, and supplementary reading materials are all useful teaching methods. Whenever possible, learning situations in which employees assume an active rather than a passive role are preferable. Use demonstrations, discussions, and role playing. Let employees assume control and learn from each other. Leadership and management development are factors to be considered. Improved education and development of supervisory personnel are becoming critical priorities in many nursing homes. With such increasing external pressures as legislation and the labor market, and with such internal pressures as employee grievances and turnover, effective supervision and management are essential. In addition, supervisors are often promoted because they are good employees or have been with the facility for a time. They may or may not have management skills. Although a training coordinator may not be asked to teach management development, he may be asked to coordinate or recommend outside training.

One basic concept to keep in mind is that training supplies specific knowledge, skills or attitudes needed by the facility. It is oriented to tasks. Management development prepares individuals to perform whole groups of tasks and to provide leadership to others. With this in mind, inservice training designed to improve the quality of patient care in nursing homes—in fact, all inservice training—would be based on the following principles from the American Hospital Association:

- All personnel must be offered the opportunity for growth, development and advancement of knowledge, understanding and skills to help them improve their on-the-job performance.
- Inservice education enables personnel to provide care and services which promote and maintain optimal levels of independent functioning among patient/residents.
- Continued improvement of the quality of inservice education serves the best interests of the nursing home, its personnel, and patient/residents.

- Continued improvement of the quality of inservice education requires active participation of representatives of all levels of personnel who are responsible for direct and indirect nursing home care and services.
- Inservice education is an integral part of the management process; the quality of inservice education practice is determined by the climate of acceptance and by appreciation and support engendered by attitudes and actions of administrative and supervisory personnel at all levels of nursing home organization.
- The climate of acceptance and appreciation of the values of inservice education is established through such administrative action as allocating monies, time, human and other resources to the inservice education program and encouraging all personnel to communicate their ideas and information about inservice education goals and processes (United Hospital Fund of New York, 1972).

A well-conducted education program that encompasses staff development, orientation, and on-the-job training is an invaluable boon to a nursing home. Such a program has the potential to save money, reduce mishaps, and increase employee satisfaction and production. The goal of this manual is to provide a resource to help develop the skills and behaviors needed to meet these goals for inservice training.

Chapter 2

Learning in an Inservice Setting

Teaching

Carl Rogers stated that it is probably impossible to teach anyone anything. Rather, the role of the effective educator is to create an environment that stimulates the desire to learn (Rogers, 1969). The responsibility to learn information must be assumed by the learner. Teaching is truly an interactive process with teachers and learners giving and receiving from one another. Teaching, like learning, is not easy; it is both an art and a science. The art is a reflection of the individual personality of the teacher and how he puts the different components together into a working whole. The science of teaching is reflected in the different techniques that teachers use to plan, present, and evaluate instruction. Teaching is based on effective decision-making—decisions regarding self, patients, learners, and the services provided.

Inservice directors are constantly deciding the who, what,

when, or how of instruction and pursuing such questions as: What am I doing here?; who are my students?; what are their learning styles?; what content/skills will be taught?; how will the information be presented?; where will the instruction take place?; when will the instruction occur?; how long will the students have to learn?; how will the students be evaluated?; are basic components of the planning process vital to inservice? Many of the critical questions may have already been decided by others. For example, subject matter may have been defined in the state or federal regulations. Facility policy may also dictate content.

The Role of an Inservice Teacher

It is difficult to list all the qualities of a good teacher. If the inservice trainer's role is to help employees learn and to create effective learning situations, many qualities will be needed. The ability to communicate ideas is essential. This encompasses the entire field of communicative skills: reading, writing, speaking, and listening. A sound philosophy of life provides the background for teaching and should also provide skill in instructional methods, including the ability to use the proper instructional technique at the right time. This leads to a need for an understanding of the way in which people learn. Basic knowledge of subject matter and the ability to learn new content is essential. An instructor should know more than those who are learning from him. Creative imagination is also a quality of an outstanding instructor, but the final, most basic quality needed is a real interest in learning. As a manager, the inservice director will also need the ability to communicate ideas; sound management philosophy; skill in organizing, recording, and monitoring; an understanding of people and their interactions; knowledge of the work environment; and a real interest in the nursing home and the people who live within it.

The above descriptions are not intended to suggest that teachers must be perfect. The point is, however, that the teacher must have a firm knowledge of himself, the subject matter to be taught, and the characteristics of the learner. Teachers are leaders, and as such they must lead. Leader behavior can create a positive climate for learning. Without it, a teacher cannot teach because learners will not learn.

Elements of Positive Leadership

Objectives need to be clearly stated at the beginning. They must be readily understandable. Learners can then be involved, either formally or informally, in the planning; their concerns can be voiced and any appropriate negotiations can be made. The teacher has the responsibility for keeping the program objective oriented, and time limited. This means that the leader's behavior must be consistent with the learning objectives; that is, he must practice what he preaches. Keeping the objectives in mind will also lend an element of predictability to the program, thus allaying anxieties some learners may have. Knowing what to expect gives one a sense of security.

Leaders need to foster a democratic atmosphere, relating equally to all the learners, not just a chosen few. During small group discussions and at break time leaders need to be available to converse with the participants. This may be an excellent time to check out feelings or to hear what shy people want to say. Language appropriate to the level of the group should be used. Any special language should be explained and used only when necessary.

The group must understand that they have some power. One way this is communicated is by taking immediate action on group decisions; another is by allowing the group to influence the content and methodology whenever possible and to renegotiate in the light of changed circumstances.

Leaders must have enough group management skills and

be sufficiently sensitive to people to handle conflict, disruptions, and passivity. Establishing an open climate will very often preclude many of these problems. By appropriate self-disclosure, the leader shows himself to be a real person with concerns, joys, and vulnerabilities like everyone else. By being warm, genuine, accepting of differences, and unthreatened by criticism, the leader builds trust in the group and fosters cooperation. Constructive feedback, rather than personal attack, will contribute to the open climate. Finally, a liberal dose of good humor will lighten sessions and promote good will. Any single inservice director may not be able to practice all these skills, but every individual can be aware of his own individual strengths and weaknesses, and can work to diminish weaknesses while building strengths.

Learning

Learning is an activity that is not restricted to a classroom or laboratory. The principles of learning carry over into the daily routine of each person's life. A person learns a given activity only by doing that activity. Learning means a change in behavior. To test the success of a training program, ask: Can the students do something they could not do before?

In addition, training is not the same thing as learning. Training is merely the administrative framework for learning. Many training programs fail because: (1) they are taught the way the person conducting the program was taught; (2) they do not clearly define a realistic objective at the beginning of the program; (3) they do not take into account the learning needs of the student.

A person cannot learn to do an activity unless the purpose of the activity is understood. A trainer cannot expect a nurse to sit in a classroom, listen to someone describe a procedure, and then be able to perform that procedure. For learning to take place, the nurse must practice in a realistic situation.

In order for a person to learn, he must want to learn. The learner's wants and needs must be considered in relation to the objectives of the program. If the program does not meet those needs the learner will not want to learn. Techniques such as role playing, small groups, and case studies help to involve the student in the learning process. These methods will be discussed in later chapters.

How much is learned depends upon the individual's ability to relate what is already known to a new situation. In other words, the degree to which a student can relate elements in a new situation to elements from a previous experience will determine the ability to learn. This principle requires individual work; each person must have the opportunity to relate the new information to what has already been learned.

The following learning principles work together to increase motivation, the rate and degree of learning, the transfer of learning to application, and the retention of information. None of these principles exists in isolation, but each contributes to the learning experience as a whole.

1. Order. Things that occur in a logical order are easier to learn than those in no order.
2. Length and complexity. Smaller amounts of information are easier to learn than large amounts. Teach segments first, then put them together to form a whole.
3. Meaning. The more meaningful the task, the easier it is to learn. Trainers must help students see meaning in what they are learning.
4. Whole versus part. The most efficient way for a student to learn is to work on the smallest segment of material that has meaning. However, overall training objectives need to be summarized first.
5. Vividness. Highlighting particular facts will draw attention to them.

6. Motivation. Possibly the most important factors in learning are the learner's willingness and interest in the material.
7. Reinforcement. Behaviors that are reinforced are more likely to be repeated than those that are not.
8. Feeling tones. If a student has a positive attitude towards the instructor and the material while learning, the learning will be more efficient.
9. Active participation. The student must be actively involved with the instructional content in order to learn.
10. Degree of guidance. Careful guidance by the trainer will greatly improve the efficiency of training and learning. Guidance should be withdrawn as the student gains proficiency.
11. Knowledge of results. A student must receive feedback if his performance is to improve. The more specific and immediate the feedback, the better.
12. Level of aspiration. The amount of material a student elects to learn over a period of time will vary from student to student.
13. Schedule of practice. Students should practice the smallest part that has maximum meaning and does not waste time. Emphasize performance, not arbitrary time limits.

The above is barely a glimpse of learning theory; volumes have been written in each of these areas. All of these factors should be considered in the planning process. One way to do this is to write a question relating to each of the above points and use these questions to evaluate the training.

Motivation

Motivation is one of the key factors in learning. If the learner is not open to the information, the teacher cannot teach. Motivation is also one of the biggest problems of inservice in nursing homes. Nurses' aides may not see any value in training. Supervisors can resent the time spent on training. Administrators may not see staff improvement. These are all motivation problems.

The basic question here is: What motivates people? This question is frequently asked and constantly researched. It is a basic concern for anyone who wishes to establish and maintain effective relations with others. It is fundamental to management and to learning. Experts agree that the following basic principles are involved in motivating others.

Rewards are a key factor in human motivation. Used appropriately, rewards reinforce behavior and motivate individuals to repeat and continue that behavior. They should always be contingent on performance; they should be personal; and they should be given as soon as possible after the observed behavior. Eliminate unnecessary threats and punishments. In the long run, positive rewards bring favorable behavior results while threats tend to have negative effects.

Allow some flexibility and provide choices. People who have been involved in the decision-making process are likely to be more motivated to follow through with the activity than those who have not. People tend to know their own capabilities and limitations and are able to set realistic goals for themselves. They are more likely to be committed to the accomplishment of goals that they have set for themselves.

Provide responsibility along with accountability. When responsibility is commensurate with a person's means, he will rarely fail to be accountable. Along with the giving of responsibility should come support. Help seeking should be encouraged and viewed as a sign of strength. In addition, the amount of supervision should reflect employees' needs, not the supervisor's needs.

Expectations for performance should be made clear. Conflicting or unclear expectations lead to frustration and ultimately to a lack of desire to perform. Providing immediate and relevant feedback will help to reinforce and clarify expectations. Good feedback gives clues to how performance might be improved, thus helping to motivate people in that direction. When criticism is in order, focus on the behavior, not the person. When possible, praise even the smallest improvements, especially when new tasks are undertaken. Giving credit whenever possible promotes a sense of accomplishment. The old saw that "nothing succeeds like success" appears to be true and is high on the list of motivators.

Arrange to get feedback from employees. When there are complaints, try to deal with them effectively and promptly. Even if the problem seems irrelevant to the task, productivity suffers when an individual's problems are ignored, and the discounted problem seems to get blown out of proportion. Handle suggestions in a democratic fashion, acknowledging appropriate input.

Exhibit interest in and knowledge of each person under supervision. This helps eliminate barriers to individual achievement and gives clues as to what rewards and reinforcers can be used effectively. People labeled as under-achievers or as poorly motivated may simply have a minor obstacle that individual attention could reveal and alleviate. Labels such as these often become self-fulfilling prophecies. Individual attention can help meet the need to feel important and personally significant.

Individuals need to participate in decisions which affect them. Motivation is inhibited by feeling powerless. At the same time the integrity, significance and relevance of one's work should be made clear in terms of the organizational purposes and goals. Finally, individual effort must pay off in results, otherwise there will be a tendency to stop trying. To a great extent, motivation is the effective management of effort.

Establishing a climate of trust and openness is vital. Trust is best encouraged by model behavior and an exhibition of confidence in other workers. Being open about one's own motivational level is often contagious. Practicing what one preaches is highly motivating to others.

Anxiety is fundamental to motivation. Although high levels of anxiety are crippling, moderate levels prevent lethargy and increase motivation. Enjoyment of a task is not always correlated with good performance. If the results of a task well done are satisfying and/or rewarded, the task itself can be boring, distasteful, or otherwise displeasing.

Short- and long-term motivation. If rewards and incentives are too remote, the motivating impact is lessened. In such cases, short-term reinforcements need to be arranged. On the other hand, if only short-term reinforcements are given, people fall short of optimum motivation, and lack a long-term perspective on their jobs. To be effective, utilize a complementary set of long- and short-term incentives and rewards.

Adult Learning

Malcolm Knowles is one of the foremost leaders in the field of adult education. He provides a number of insights into adult learning (Knowles, 1970). Adults have at least four characteristics as learners that differ from those of youth as learners (especially as typically assumed in traditional schooling).

Self-concept. Youth tend to see themselves as essentially dependent persons. They enter an educational activity with the concept that their role is the more or less passive one of receiving information adults have decided they should have.

Adults, on the other hand, tend to see themselves as responsible, self-directing, independent personalities. Adults have a deep psychological need to be treated with respect, to be perceived as self-sufficient. They tend to avoid, resist, and resent being placed in situations in which they feel they are treated like children; that is, situations in which they are told what to do and what not to do, talked down to, embarrassed, punished, or judged. Knowles (1970) suggests the following advice for adult educators.

1. Create a climate of mutual respect, of warmth and informality, of freedom from threat and judgment, of positive regard for each person.
2. Use procedures that let the learner deeply and objectively diagnose his own needs for learning rather than let the trainer diagnose the student's needs.
3. Involve the students in the learning process. Mutually formulate objectives and design learning activities.
4. Share responsibility with the students for actually conducting the learning activity.
5. Use procedures that let learners evaluate their own progress toward learning goals.
6. Shift the trainer's role from that of director and transmitter of learning to that of stimulator and resource for self-inquiry.

Amount of experience.   A typical adult, simply by having lived longer than a typical youth, enters into an educational activity with a greater volume of experience. Therefore, adult learners are usually a richer resource for learning than are youth; they are less dependent on the vicarious experiences of teachers, experts, and textbooks; they have a broader foundation of information on which to base new ideas. On the other hand, they may also have more fixed habits of thought. Knowles (1970) gives us the following points regarding experience:

1. Emphasize experiential techniques such as discussion, case method, and simulation. Down play such methods as lecture, assigned reading, quizzes, and audio-visual presentations.

2. Examine the relationship between new concepts and the life experiences of the students.
3. Open up habit patterns with preliminary unfreezing activities such as feedback exercises.

Readiness to learn.   Youth resist learning things that are not specifically related to the developmental tasks at each stage of growth. Adults, too, are most ready to learn those things required by the developmental tasks of their current stage of growth be it early adulthood, middle age, or later maturity. Again Knowles (1970) advises:

1. The developmental tasks of a particular group of learners provide a better guide for determining the sequence of learning activities than the logical needs of an institution or subject matter expert.
2. Motivation will be increased if ways can be found to help adults become more aware of their developmental task.

Developmental tasks evolve out of the changing requirements of the social roles of adulthood. For example, in the role of worker the first developmental task is to get a job; at that point, one is ready to learn anything required to get a job but not much else about the worker role. That is, one is not ready to learn about supervising others on the job until the job itself has first been mastered and the getting ahead phase is entered.

Time perspective.   Youth tend to perceive most of their learning as being useful for later life, with postponed application influencing their time perspective. Their orientation to learning is that of accumulating subject-matter knowledge. Adults, on the other hand, engage in learning largely in response to pressures they feel from current life problems. They hope to get some help in dealing more adequately with situations they are experiencing in the present. Their time perspective is one of immediate application, and their orientation to learning is that of problem solving.

Youth tend to be subject-centered in their approach to learning; adults are problem-centered. In response to this issue Knowles (1970) prescribes the following:

1. Units of learning that are organized around the life problems of the learners will be perceived as being more relevant than units organized by subject matter.
2. Programs based on information from the students about the problems they want help with are more likely to be effective than other programs.
3. Descriptions of learning units that are problem oriented will be perceived as being more relevant than those that are subject-oriented.

In light of these differences an educator will want to work to create a learning atmosphere in which learning is a cooperative effort and the trainer is not the only teacher. Incorporating feedback from on-the-job application of training will lessen the feeling of dependency learners may have. Utilizing nonlecture teaching techniques also promotes learner involvement. A good training coordinator will facilitate the getting ahead phase in a worker's hierarchy of developmental tasks. This phase may entail supervising new employees during orientation, helping with teaching, demonstrating, or contemplating career advancement. Good training should facilitate these objectives.

Occasionally the planned training session will need to be scrapped or modified in response to immediate problems which need to be solved. A crisis on the floor is far more important to the learners than the subject of a standard lesson plan. Also, when a problem arises for which no possible solution is to be found within the training context, it may be even more important to devote some time to the airing of feelings and the sharing of opinions. Staying tuned in to these differences in adult learners will enhance a trainer's effectiveness.

Anxiety

Most adults experience some anxiety in the classroom. This is often expressed as hostility, refusal to interact, or a demand for attention. One way to overcome this is to begin each training with a "getting to know you" interchange. The trainer should introduce himself and mention personal facts about background and qualifications. Adults react more positively to qualified teachers. Cohesiveness is engendered by encouraging interchange. Physical arrangements should be comfortable and should promote interaction.

The trainer should assure the group that any contribution or question is welcome; participation should be encouraged using positive reinforcement. Positive reactions to comments and questions is one way to foster group participation in adults. For example, a trainer might say, "That is a good question because. . . ." Never ignore a comment or question no matter how trite or negative it might be. The trainer should understand that the learners come from diverse backgrounds. A learner cannot be forced to participate. Do not become impatient if directions must be repeated.

A trainer should never read material. Rather, he should learn facts and use a comfortable delivery style. A trainer at ease will enable the learners to be at ease.

Memory

When the inservice requires memorization, the inservice director can be helpful in many ways. Cuing redundantly and using oral and written presentations, writing on the chalkboard as the words are being said, and encouraging note taking are some ways of aiding memory. Requesting definitions from the group and avoiding jargon except when it is a necessary part of the instruction also help. The trainer should not do all the talking. Encourage the group to verbalize concepts. Whenever possible, illustrate concepts by sharing personal experiences that can serve as examples of the ideas that are being taught. Encouraging students to relate their experience to classroom concepts will aid learning and encourage individual thinking and participation.

In summary, by learning from the students, organizing presentations carefully and efficiently, using time wisely, and developing empathy for adult learners, the inservice trainer will be likely to direct a successful training program.

When teaching nursing home employees, it is important to remember that it has been a long time since some of the students have attended a class. Assume that they feel some uneasiness and insecurity. Their feelings could stop them from listening and learning new skills. It is critical that specific objectives are clearly stated at the onset of each class; also exact expectations of learners should be stated.

Some students may have negative ideas about classes, education, or even learning new ideas. They may associate classes with past experiences that were failures. Typical thoughts that these students may have are: "This is stupid. Why do I have to be here?" "What does this have to do with my job?" "Will I lose my job if I don't do well in this class?" An inservice director should tune in to those unsaid statements. Rephrase the statements positively; for example, "How do you think this could help employees on the job?"

Some students may worry about looking foolish in front of their peers. Also, they may sense some competition with their peers. One useful technique in these situations is to involve all learners in planning and instruction.

Each learner is unique and has his own learning style. For example, some students may prefer reading information for themselves rather than attending sessions; they may be independent learners. Some students may learn better by discussing information with co-workers; they may be collaborative learners. Some students may be motivated to learn by sheer competition; for these students a rewards system with positive consequences for all involved is needed. There are general patterns of learning styles and an array of teaching methods designed to meet the individual needs and the needs of specific facilities.

Classroom Management/Group Control

Although understanding the adult learner is vitally important and adequate preparation is essential, these factors alone cannot ensure successful training. The trainer must know how to effectively manage a group of students. Group control is not manipulative or autocratic domination. Rather, it involves managing a group to provide an efficient atmosphere for learning. Effective management is critical to effective instruction. Educational researchers have verified a relationship between trainers who are effective classroom managers and students who achieve well and have good attitudes about learning.

No one best approach to classroom management and group control has been found. This section looks at a few problems adult learners may have in the classroom, and examines several suggestions for effective group control. Each person has a fundamental need to feel worthwhile and to belong. If a student is frustrated in fulfilling his needs in socially acceptable ways, inappropriate behavior such as seeking attention, seeking power, seeking revenge, and/or showing inadequacy or helplessness may be displayed. In adult learners these behaviors show up in a variety of ways, such as sleeping in class, arguing every point, not listening, asking antagonistic questions, or acting generally non-responsive.

Problems in the classroom are also related to group interaction. Several problems pertaining to adult learning that have been identified are: lack of unity; ignoring of established norms; negative reactions to individuals; distraction or stopping of work; resistance to the trainer; and resistance to change in the working environment. Examples of these behaviors include: taking sides; talkative behavior; ridicule of a group member; and hostile and aggressive attitudes. In light of these potentially disruptive classroom situations, trainers need to have a good understanding of group control and how to use it in order to make learning more effective.

The two methods of group control to be avoided are authoritarianism and permissiveness. An authoritarian trainer views classroom management as a matter of controlling the student. The trainer establishes and maintains order by dominating students. This is a dehumanizing approach for learners. In contrast, in a permissive situation the trainer has a laissez-faire attitude. The trainer maximizes student freedom by allowing students free rein in the classroom. This approach is unrealistic in that training goals are seldom attained.

An effective trainer will want to incorporate various characteristics of effective teaching and learning into an overall picture of classroom management. A trainer can increase the effectiveness of learning while realistically controlling the group by building interpersonal relationships and by being genuine. A person with whom the students can relate establishes a comfortable atmosphere in which adults are better able to learn. The trainer should also accept the students as trustworthy and should show confidence in their abilities. Try to understand the students from their point of view and try to be constantly aware of feelings. If a difficulty arises, talk to the situation rather than to the personality or character. Always avoid sarcasm, preaching, and nagging, and avoid demands and commands; instead use appreciative praise and encourage students to express their ideas and feelings. By establishing a democratic classroom through regular, frank discussions that foster mutual trust, the trainer will allow each student to learn at maximum capacity.

Six characteristics of effective classroom management have been identified.

1. Expectations are individual predictions of the way in which people will behave in a group setting. They influence the relationship between the trainer and the student. In an effective classroom expectations are accurate, realistic, and clearly understood. A trainer will need to identify his own expectations and those of the learners. Some reconciliations may need to occur.
2. Leadership involves the behaviors that lead a group to its objectives. In an effective classroom, both students and trainer show leadership behaviors. Leadership functions should be well distributed, and all group members should feel self-worth in working together. Students who share leadership responsibility with the trainer are more likely to be responsible for their own behavior. The effective trainer creates a climate in which students can be leaders.
3. Attraction refers to the friendship patterns in the classroom group. The effective trainer fosters interpersonal relationships among group members while avoiding the formation of destructive cliques.
4. Norms are shared expectations of the way group members should think, feel, and behave. They provide a frame of reference to guide the students' behaviors. The group

regulates behavior by exerting pressure on members to adhere to the norms. The effective trainer helps the group set up productive norms.

5. Communication means the receiver correctly interprets the message that the sender intends to deliver. The effective trainer opens channels of communication so all students express their thoughts and feelings freely.

6. Cohesiveness emphasizes the individual's relationship to the group as a whole. The effective trainer encourages cohesiveness through promoting the previously discussed properties, thus making group membership both attractive and satisfying.

Understanding why people behave the way they do can help make an effective training session. Consider the following common group management problems and the suggestions for their elimination:

1. Avoidance of the task. Frequently, when a group dodges the main issue, something is keeping the members from real work. They may feel overwhelmed by the issues; they may feel inadequate to deal with the material; they may lack the desire to work hard; they may feel hostility toward the trainer; or they may have other, more pressing needs. The trainer may have to remind the group that they are avoiding the task. Learners should begin to take responsibility for their own behavior.

2. Members' impatience with each other. When a group is on edge, members speak more vehemently, and subtle personal attacks creep in. Possible causes include the group's dissatisfaction with itself and resentment toward the trainer. The group should be urged to focus on the learning task, not on personalities or other personal issues.

3. Ideas attacked before full expression. Statements frequently are attacked before the speaker has finished; every sug-

gestion is viewed as impractical; no one listens fully to others; cliques are formed. If emotions are high, the trainer may suggest that a speaker at least be asked if he is finished. The trainer may also paraphrase what was said so that the speaker knows he was heard.

4. Inactive listening. Body language provides many clues. Students may be yawning with boredom or leaning forward intently, waiting to break in with their own contributions. Facial expressions may signal danger. Trainers may find out that when they are actively listening, other members of the group will follow suit.

Summary

Effective classroom management is a product of the trainer's good leadership and realistic expectations. In addition, the trainer must understand normal group dynamics and be alert to symptoms of problem situations. Effective training requires an understanding of the individual person, the manner in which that person learns, the group, and the intra- and inter-relations of the group. The trainer must be part of the group, in control of the group, and outside of the group watching for changes. It is a difficult job.

Chapter 3
Planning, Needs Assessment, and Objectives

Planning

Thorough planning is no guarantee that an uneventful training session will suddenly change into a stimulating one, but it will give the inservice a direction and an outline that could make the difference between the learner's being bored or being benefited. Planning is an essential skill in training because it incorporates all areas of the learning process from developing behavioral objectives and assessing students' needs to deciding the presentation mode and evaluating course material. While some inservice directors look upon planning as drudgery, others view it as a teaching aid and an invaluable organizational boon. This chapter presents and explains the advantages of planning and the ways it can be used to improve the effectiveness of a trainer's lesson presentation.

Inservice education is like a giant crossword puzzle. With time, trial and error, and patience, the major pieces fit together to form a whole. There are many models an inservice director can follow to design the actual training sessions. The model shown in Figure 3.1 is most often followed and appears to have the most flexibility for planning. It is a circular model with six major components: needs analysis; identification of instructional content; establishment of goals and objectives; delivery of training; evaluation of learning; and revision of plans to more fully meet intended outcomes.

Needs Analysis

Needs analysis is a process of defining the desired outcomes of a training program. It is a logical problem-solving tool used to specify what the content of training should be and what trainees should be able to do. The basic question of a needs analysis

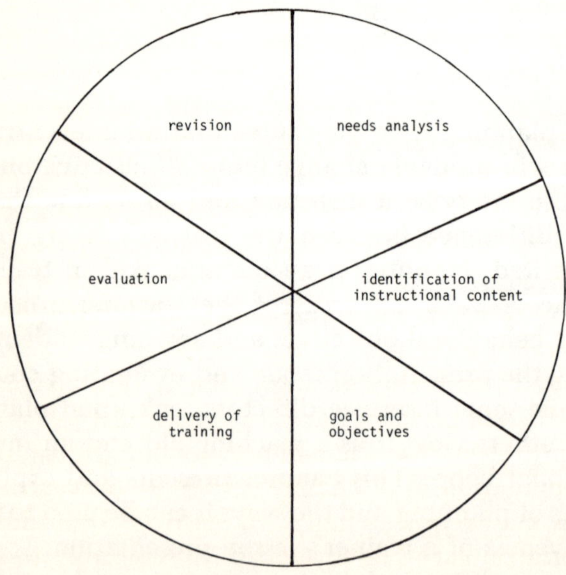

Figure 3.1.   Flexible Planning Model

is: Does the employee know how to meet the performance standards for the job he is to perform? If the answer to the question is yes, then no training is needed. However, if the answer is no, training is needed.

Sometimes the answer to the question is yes, but the employee, for a variety of reasons, does not perform his job. This is a management, not a training problem. Inservice may help to alleviate these kinds of problems by using programs that deal with feelings and management/employee relations; but inservice alone cannot solve them.

The process of needs analysis can be represented by the following formula: desired performance minus actual performance equals training need. This is a basic discrepancy model. The first step is to identify the desired levels of employee performance. The second step is to measure actual performance. If there is a difference between the desired level and the actual level, adjustments in performance must be made.

Desired levels of employee performance can be identified in a number of ways. The first step in the process is the job of the nursing home administrator. The administrator, with the staff, must decide what knowledge, skills, and attitudes employees must have in order to perform their jobs according to minimum standards. This step can be accomplished by reviewing current job descriptions, reviewing state and/or federal standards, and by observing current employees who are judged competent. These employees can be asked to keep a diary or log of work roles and can provide valuable aid in listing job criteria for the various positions.

Changes within the nursing home or new developments within the field of geriatric care may also affect job standards. The administration may change policies and procedures. The resident population may change in needs. New government regulations may require change in staffing. In addition, the field of geriatric care has expanded considerably in the past few years, and recent developments can be excellent training topics.

The second step is to measure actual employee performance. The two best ways to do this are to observe and to ask. The inservice director should be a familiar figure in the nursing home and should observe employee performance at all levels. Checklists and observation sheets of desired behaviors should be developed; supervisors should be asked to observe employees. Employees should observe their own work behaviors and measure them against the established standards. Employees themselves often know what skills they need to develop but do not know how to learn them or who to ask for additional training. Positive communication between employees and the inservice director can develop a climate of trust in which employees know that needs will be met in a nonthreatening manner. Residents, families, and other employees should be talked to, with consideration and tact for individual differences and feelings; observation and self-report can provide an accurate picture of employee competency.

Once a discrepancy between existing performance and desired performance is agreed upon, there are three major ways of reducing the discrepancy. The first is by training the employees in new behaviors, skills, and attitudes, and changing those that exist and are undesirable. The second is to change the environmental conditions. Rearranging materials or equipment, relocating residents or personnel, or establishing different procedures can affect employee performance. The third is to redefine values; expectations, goals, policies, or priorities may need to be revised so that conditions fall within tolerance levels.

Training is not always the best solution to reducing discrepancies. It must be determined that training can solve the problem before the inservice trainer continues through the planning steps.

Following is an example. The director of nurses has been able to persuade the administrator of a nursing home that the ratio of aides to patients on the afternoon shift needs to be increased. This will enable the schedule of patient care activities (baths, for example) to be more flexible. That is, it will no longer be necessary for the 7 to 3 shift to complete all the routine patient care now required. This change in staffing and procedures has worked well for the morning shift since they were continually overloaded and unable to complete assigned duties. It also fits well with the social activities. However, there have been complaints from the enlarged afternoon shift that patients' naps and favorite television programs, plus regular bedtime routines, still prohibit absorbing the extra duties assigned. (The afternoon aides perceive these extra duties as unnecessarily time consuming and burdensome.) Relatives, too, have been objecting to finding patients involved in care procedures at hours when they prefer to visit.

The solutions to this problem may be:

- Training people. The afternoon aides may need to review certain patient care activities that they have not been previously responsible for.
- Changing environmental conditions. Some rescheduling of staff has occurred and the greater flexibility in patient care activities has resulted in more effective use of the facilities, that is, fewer residents being bathed in one time span. Therefore, bathing is more relaxed and can be a pleasurable activity.
- Redefining values. Training will include attitudinal material aimed at emphasizing that excellent patient care is the goal of the facility and should be flexible to meet the needs of patients, not those of staff and family.

This problem, then, can be solved through training. The training director can schedule a program which may include a review and practice of patient care activities, and/or a simulation of patient care activities in which emphasis is placed on the patients' social and psychological needs.

Once it has been decided that a training need does exist, the trainer should look at the level of need. There are various levels of training needs. Micro-needs involve only one person while macro-needs are high priority needs that demand continuous attention. Macro-needs can be met within an ongoing, continuous inservice system that, once established, can be repeated as needed. An example of this is orientation. Once the inservice director has established the needed parts of a workable orientation and has developed the materials (for example, orientation manuals) and procedure, other personnel within the home can be responsible for teaching this session on a regular basis. Micro-needs are individual. They are dealt with in one session on a one to one basis. For example, a nurse on wing two may notice one of the aides lifting and transferring patients incorrectly. The inservice director would demonstrate the correct procedure to that aide and follow through with review and practice until the aide could perform the procedures correctly. Another example of a micro-need would be initial training of personnel when new equipment is purchased. All personnel to be involved with the use of the new equipment would need to be trained for its operation and maintenance, and this new information would then have to be incorporated into orientation. But after the initial training has been completed, it should not have to be repeated.

Measurement is crucial in the needs analysis process. Measurement can be used to determine both desired level of employee performance and current level of performance. Measurement can be defined as the gathering of objective data and is usually done by observing behavior on a formal or an informal basis.

Data concerning training needs can come from a variety of sources. Some of these sources are:

promotions	new equipment
transfers	new procedures
appraisals	changes in regulations, standards

accidents

quality control

grievances

new positions

special assignments

job descriptions

cross-qualification of
employees

new policies

key requests, reports

supervisors

employees

residents

families

new trends in the nursing home
field

The trainer can also use a variety of methods for collecting data. Some of these methods are interviews, questionnaires, job analysis, records and reports, and group analysis procedures. Figure 3.2 lists some of the advantages and disadvantages of these methods.

One of the most popular ways to conduct a needs assessment in a nursing home is to develop a short rating scale for supervisors. Below is an example of one that could be used to rate nurse aides on skills relating to taking and recording vital signs.

Directions: Please rate each of your aides on the following tasks.

Task	Performs very well				Performs poorly
	1	2	3	4	5
1. Choose correct type of thermometer (rectal/oral)	___	___	___	___	___
2. Observe proper care of thermometer	___	___	___	___	___
3. Take an oral temperature using correct procedures	___	___	___	___	___
4. Take a rectal temperature using correct procedures	___	___	___	___	___
5. Record temperature correctly	___	___	___	___	___

METHOD	ADVANTAGES	LIMITATIONS	DO'S AND DONT'S
Interviews	Reveals feelings, causes and possible solutions of problems as well as facts.	Is time consuming.	Pretest and revise interview questions as needed.
	Affords maximum opportunity for free expression of opinion, giving of suggestions.	Can make subject feel she/he is "on the spot."	Be sure interviewer can and does listen, doesn't judge responses.
Questionnaire	Can reach many people in short time.	Little provision for free expression of unanticipated responses	Pretest; revise questions and form as needed.
	Is relatively inexpensive.	May be difficult to construct.	Offer and safeguard anonymity.
	Gives opportunity of expression without fear of embarrassment.	Has limited effectiveness in getting at causes of problems and possible solutions.	Use only if prepared to report both favorable and unfavorable findings and do something about them.
	Yields data easily. Can be summarized and reported easily.		
Job Analysis and Performance Review	Produces specific and precise information about jobs and performance.	Time consuming	Be sure analysis is of current job and current performance.
	Is directly tied to actual jobs and to on-the-job performance	Difficult for people not specifically trained in job analysis techniques.	Review with employees both analysis of job and appraisal of performance.

	Breaks job into segments manageable both for training and for appraisal purposes.	Supervisors often dislike reviewing employees' inadequacies with them personally. Reveals training needs of individuals but not those based on needs of organization.	
Records and Reports Study	Provides excellent clues to trouble spots. Provides objective evidence of results Are usually of concern to **and ea**sily understood by administration	Does not show causes of problems, or possible solutions. May not reflect current situation, recent changes.	Use as checks and clues, in combination with other methods.
Group Problem Analysis	Permits synthesis of different viewpoints. Promotes general understanding and agreement. Builds support for needed training. Is in itself good training.	Is time consuming and initially expensive. Supervisors may feel too busy to participate, want work done for them.	Do not promise or expect quick results. Identify all problems of significant concern to group and start with one of those identified. Let group make own analysis, set own priorities.

Figure 3.2.   Methods of Determining Needs

The head nurse on one of the wings rated twelve of her aides in the following manner.

Task	Number of responses				
1. Choose correct type of thermometer (rectal/oral)	10	2	0	0	0
2. Observe proper care of thermometer	9	3	0	0	0
3. Take an oral temperature using correct procedures	12	0	0	0	0
4. Take a rectal temperature using correct procedures	6	3	3	0	0
5. Record temperature correctly	4	3	2	3	0

What does the above mean for the inservice trainer? Obviously, tasks 1, 2, and 3 are being performed well. Task 4 could use some review during the next inservice as only six of the twelve aides are performing very well in this area. Task 5 is a high training priority. Training on correctly recording temperatures needs to be implemented immediately.

Needs analysis is an essential part of the planning process. Through needs analysis the trainer can determine who needs training, what level of training is needed, and what the content of the training should include. Once the trainer comes up with several broad ideas or concepts for the training session, students should be given a chance to review those concepts and offer suggestions. Involving the students in this phase of planning can motivate them to learn.

From these general concepts evolves a teaching unit—a specific plan of action for the learning sessions. A content outline is helpful at this point; it should be detailed enough to indicate points of emphasis. The trainer can use this outline as the basis for developing instructional objectives.

Instructional Objectives

A teaching plan that does not focus on one or more instructional objectives is, at best, directionless. Without a specific goal or objective in mind, a trainer will find that little is accomplished.

According to Mager (1975, p. 3), an objective is "an intent communicated by a statement describing a proposed change in a learner—a statement of what the learner is to be like when he has successfully completed a learning experience."

The following are examples of acceptable learning objectives:

- By the end of the training period, the learner will be able to write three examples of how to communicate with residents who need reality orientation therapy.
- After hearing the lecture on changes in visual processes and aging, the learner will be able to list the changes that occur.
- The student will be able to complete a client intake assessment from a taped interview. The lower limit of acceptable performance will be 38 of 45 items answered correctly within an examination period of 90 minutes.
- The student will be able to write a description of the steps involved in taking vital signs.
- The student must be able to correctly name each department within the facility and state the basic function of each.

Objectives, therefore, should reflect what the student rather than the teacher will do.

Although deciding and writing behavioral objectives can be a chore, the benefits are many. Objectives form the framework for any instructional program in which mastery of learning is the desired outcome. Objectives inform learners of what will be required of them, and they help the planner to think in specific terms. They provide the best means for communicating to others what is to be taught and learned. The type and extent of activities that are required for successfully carrying out the learning are indicated by the type and extent of the objectives. Organizing and sequencing the subject matter is easier when objectives are defined. Objectives provide a basis for evaluating both the learning and the effectiveness of the program.

An instructional objective is a statement that describes an intended outcome of instruction; it should never be merely a description or summary of content; it should be stated in performance terms that describe what the learner will be doing when he demonstrates achievement of the objective; it should communicate an instructional intent to a reader, and do so to the degree that it describes or defines the terminal behavior expected of the learner.

To describe terminal behavior (what the learner will be doing):

1. Identify and name the overall behavior act.
2. Define the important conditions under which the behavior is to occur (for example, time limit).
3. Define the criterion of acceptable performance (for example, student must answer 16 of 20 questions correctly).

The statement of objectives for an entire program of instruction will consist of several specific statements, not one broad, encompassing statement. The objective that is most usefully stated is one that best communicates the instructional intent of the person selecting the objective (Mager, 1975).

An objective communicates the trainer's intent to the degree that it describes what the learner will be doing when demonstrating achievement, and how the trainer will know when the achievement occurs. After writing objectives, always check to see that they reflect what the student will be doing rather than what the trainer will do. Write a separate statement for each objective; the more statements the better the chance of making intent clear.

The next step in developing learning objectives is to give each learner a copy of the objectives. Once the learner is acquainted with the objectives, he can participate in the learning in a responsible fashion. Knowing what is expected in the learning situation, learners can monitor their own progress and request clarification, repetition, or review of material in line with stated objectives. In this manner, the learner becomes responsible for his own learning.

An example that demonstrates the use of instructional objectives in a nursing home setting is presented below. An inservice for nurses' aides in appropriate methods for taking patients' vital signs is being developed. The instructional objectives should describe educational intents (goals). In this case, the intent is to teach aides techniques for taking vital signs—including oral temperature, rectal temperature, pulse, respiration, and blood pressure. Since objectives should describe what the learner will be doing when demonstrating achievement of this goal, the objectives will need to describe such behavior. As previously mentioned, the description will need to be in terms of: (1) the behavior itself; (2) the conditions under which the behavior is to occur; and (3) the criterion of acceptance of the behavior. In the following examples of objectives, each of these three parts is identified.

- By the end of this inservice training (condition, 2), aides will be able to demonstrate the correct method (criterion of acceptance, 3) of taking oral temperature (terminal behavior, 1).
- By the end of this inservice training (2), aides will be able to write three valid reasons (3) for using a rectal thermometer instead of an oral thermometer (1).
- After watching a demonstration on how to take the pulse

rate (2), aides will be able to write instructions (3) for this procedure (1).

- After three trials (2), the aide will be able to demonstrate taking another person's blood pressure (1), correctly describing the process involved (3).
- Given a sample of vital signs (2), the aide will be able to record the information (1) in proper form in the temperature, pulse rate, and respiration (TPR) notebook (3).

These examples are simply suggestions designed for the purpose of illustrating how to construct educational objectives; they may not be appropriate for any one particular inservice. However, the behavior of aides completing the training has been described (all #1 phrases), the conditions under which it will occur have been stipulated (all #2 phrases), and the acceptable levels of performance have been identified (all #3 phrases). Evaluation of achievement of these objectives will indicate how well the training reached its goal of teaching techniques for obtaining vital signs.

In summary, an instructional objective is a clear statement describing a proposed change in a learner. Objectives provide the trainer with a sound basis for planning instructional and evaluation procedures. Objectives provide the learner with the knowledge of what is to be learned; they are the roadmaps of learning.

Planning for teaching is a flexible process. There is an interdependence among the parts. Decisions relating to one part can and will affect the others. Ideally one should start with the needs analysis, but in reality that may not be possible. Start with whatever element is possible and move backward and forward until all the elements have been considered. Then rework and revise. Planning for teaching is a constant process.

Inservice Session Plans

Plans are not made to be broken, just revised. An argument that some inservice directors give for not writing lesson plans is that a teacher needs to feel free to react spontaneously as instructional opportunities arise. The results of a California study (Cooper et al., 1977) show, however, that few teachers actually made drastic changes in planned lessons once they were under way, regardless of whether or not the original plans were written out in detail or were simply mental notes. Teachers did make adjustments in their plans, but for the most part those adjustments were small procedural refinements. This indicates that teachers are not as flexible as some would indicate. All teachers plan; therefore good planning is the backbone of good inservice teaching. The plan should be written down. The best plan is one that everyone can see and follow. The lesson plan that follows (Table 3.1) is included as an example of a system of writing lesson plans.

Good plans are often shared. Many plans are available in curriculum guidelines and prepared materials. There is value in reviewing good plans previously used. They can form the basis for creative inservice and can broaden the inservice directors' list of possible topics and resources.

Do planners make better teachers? The Cooper study looked for relationships between the kinds of planning teachers did and the average amount of learning students achieved in special two week units. No simple relationships were found. The study did, however, indicate that teachers whose students learned more made fewer general statements in their lesson plans. That is, their statements tended to be specific.

The process of planning begins when a teacher or trainer determines what major ideas or dimensions he wishes to emphasize over a selected period of time. All available instructional materials should be gathered and reviewed at this time.

Table 3.1. Sample Lesson Plan

Course: Orientation to Patient Care   *Class:* Taking Temperatures   *Time:* 1 hour
Facility: Inservice classroom   *Media:* Large thermometer chart, inservice dummy
Equipment: Thermometers (oral/rectal), cotton, alcohol, pencils, paper

Objectives	Content	Learning Activities	Evaluation
Students will be able to choose correct type of thermometer (oral/rectal).	Importance of temperature: when, where, why, how	State objectives; short lecture and demonstration	5 item paper test
Students will be able to demonstrate proper care of thermometer.	Procedure for care: storage, handling, cleaning	Demonstration	Student demonstration
Students will be able to take oral temperature, using correct procedures.	Procedure for oral temperature	Demonstration (student volunteer)	Student demonstration, using another student
Students will be able to take rectal temperature, using correct procedures.	Procedure for rectal temperature	Demonstration (dummy)	Student demonstration, using dummy
Students will be able to record temperature correctly.	Procedure for recording	Lecture (thermometer chart)	10 item paper test

Relying on a single text or reference is not a good idea; it makes the trainer and learners slaves to a single frame of reference.

In summary, planning decisions should be both simple and complex, both long-range and short-term; the basic points remain the same.

1. Planning helps the learner to become an active participant in the teaching/learning process.
2. Planning provides explicit directions for learning.
3. Planning helps structure the learning session so that it proceeds from simple to complex activities.
4. Needs assessment, as part of overall planning, measures the learner's prior knowledge so that learning can begin where appropriate. Learning should start from where the learner is, both educationally and experientially, and proceed accordingly.
5. Planning can help the inservice director ensure a variety of learning activities; these include seeing, doing, hearing, speaking, and writing.
6. Planning provides a basic structure around which specific class activities are organized as well as providing a long-range guide for future sessions.

Summary

Time spent on planning, conducting an assessment of learner needs and organizational needs, and writing behavioral objectives sometimes appears wasted. One has a temptation to skip these steps and proceed directly to teaching. However, that time is not wasted, for without adequate plans and measurement of actual needs, there is no way to know whether the training itself was entertaining, but directionless—or useful and needed.

Chapter 4

Lecture, Demonstration, and Discussion

Of all the teaching methods available to trainers, lecture, demonstration, and discussion are the most successful and frequently used. They can also be the least successful and most often abused methods. Each of these inservice methods is economical because each allows the trainer to present information or demonstrate skills to many people at once. The issue of economy is important. A one-time lecture to a group of students in one room is less expensive and more efficient than a method that involves many groups in several rooms at different times.

The trainer should consider each seriously before deciding that the information should be delivered via any one particular method. Each has limitations as well as advantages. A trainer should make certain that the goal for a particular session is well suited to one teaching method rather than to another method, before he decides to use the technique. Too often trainers use lecture, demonstration, or discussion because other possible methods have not been explored, because the material has always been presented using these approaches, or because they were trained using these methods.

The following discussion is included to help facilitate the making of informed decisions concerning choice of presentation.

Lecture

There are many advantages to using the lecture technique. The trainer who chooses this method will convey information to the audience by providing an overview of the material to be covered, by providing information in a listening format, and by transmitting the information in an organized and concise manner. Lecture can provide a large amount of information in a short period of time to a large audience. Opinions and information can be presented with a minimum of cost or delay.

However, most people do not learn best by auditory means, and they may be easily distracted during a lecture. Adding visual aids will enhance the effectiveness of the lecture method of presentation. Holding the lecture to fifteen to twenty minute segments will also improve learning.

Use of lecture allows information to be transmitted to people who cannot read. Educational aids, such as films and charts, can be easily incorporated into the lecture. Speakers can present up-to-date information such as works in progress and recent research not otherwise available. Many adults have had experience with this form of teaching and will feel relatively comfortable.

However, there are some limitations to lecturing. Only one person's ideas can be presented. This often results in a rather limited scope. The lecture provides only a low level of stimulation for the learners; the audience has no opportunity for verbal participation. Facts may be inaccurate or distorted by a careless or poorly prepared speaker. The speaker may have difficulty making provisions for differences in his audience's backgrounds and learning styles. Speakers generally present material relevant to only a small portion of the audience. Speakers may be more concerned about their own performance than the audience's grasp of the material. Learners can become tired or bored if the speaker goes on too long, talks on an inappropriate level, or does not have a pleasant manner of speaking.

Should the lecture method be chosen, careful preparation must be undertaken. A lecture can add up to nothing more than wasted time if it is not thoroughly researched and planned. An effective lecture will reflect the following considerations.

1. Clear decisions as to the purpose of the lecture should be made and objectives stated. The lecture should fit the context of information that has come before and information that will follow. The presenter must become familiar with the material to be presented in relation to what the learners already know.
2. Careful research is essential. Notes of any new information to be included, as well as any specific facts or figures, should be made. Also, media, such as tapes and filmstrips, should be prepared well in advance. A variety of media makes for a diverse and more interesting lecture. The educational level, background, and interest of the audience should be discovered and a vocabulary compatible with that of the audience chosen.
3. The lecture should be planned to fit the allotted time with time for a question period. Also the room and needed equipment should be scheduled in advance, the equipment supplied and usable. Everyone should be able to see and hear the lecturer.
4. An effective lecturer should consider a succinct and smooth presentation essential to reaching the objectives. The lecturer must not only transmit information to the audience,

but also must motivate listeners to further study. This can be accomplished by grabbing the attention of the audience through the use of humor, illustrations, and personal examples.

5. Clarifying the objectives for the audience will allow learners to listen more attentively because they know the trainer's goal. An outline for the audience to follow which places the lecture topic in the context of what the audience already knows gives the students a focus for their attention.

6. The presentation style also helps to keep audience attention. The presentation should be paced to suit both the objectives of the lecture and the ability of the students, allowing plenty of time for note taking. Monotonous and pompous presentations should be avoided, questions invited. Everyone learns better when actively involved. The main points of the lecture should be reviewed at the end and a brief summary provided. This will aid listeners in conceptualizing the content and will provide an immediate review of basic points.

7. The introduction to the lecture can serve such functions as establishing rapport with learners and gaining attention. The content should be relevant to the interests and needs of the learners and should provide motivational cues. The introduction should also expose essential content in a preliminary way, based on predetermined objectives; it should remind learners of related ideas they already know. It should introduce the objectives for the presentation.

8. The body of the lecture—the content—should be clear and explicit, making use of patterns, links, verbal markers of importance, and structural supports. To maintain attention during the lecture, stimuli may be varied and communication channels changed. Physical activity, such as letting learners move around the room, also helps to hold attention. Enthusiasm in all its forms is almost sure

to help learners learn more. Inserting questions into the lecture also has been shown to have good effects.

9. The conclusion should summarize what learners should now know and be able to do. The trainer's expression of thanks for the audience's attention has been found to be related to greater learning. Asking questions gives all participants a final opportunity to clarify certain points. Reviewing the way in which this lecture is related to previous and subsequent learning and the way in which the material presented can be used within the learners' job roles is an excellent way of finalizing the presentation.

Demonstration

Demonstrations help to translate knowledge or theory into teaching practice. The carefully prepared demonstration, accompanied by oral and visual explanation, is an efficient way to teach a procedure or technique to a group. Most demonstrations allow time for the learners to practice the new procedure under the guidance of the presenter. Learning will increase, because the learners are able to listen as well as do and see. The instructor can make an instant evaluation when the learner is allowed to make a return demonstration. There are several advantages to giving a demonstration. A procedure or skill can be clarified more easily than it can when it is presented verbally. Learning is enhanced through clear, vivid demonstration of a procedure's steps and key points. The learner can practice opportunities under guidance. Errors can be corrected immediately. The use of things can be taught more readily via demonstration.

Demonstrations do, however, have limitations. The group may be too large for everyone to practice what has been demonstrated. Only practical, not abstract, skills can be demonstrated. It may be difficult for all students to see and hear the demonstration. A poorly performed demonstration may bring about unfavorable reactions from the audience. As with the lecture method, an informative demonstration is inefficient without proper planning and research. The demonstration is most effective when every detail is planned, precise, and smooth. Trainers should incorporate the steps outlined above in discussing preparation of a lecture into planning a demonstration.

In addition, the trainer will also have to incorporate the following points into the planning. A specific goal or purpose for the demonstration must be defined. The skill the learners should be able to perform after the demonstration must be clearly analyzed and defined in detail.

Tools and equipment needed for the demonstration should be collected in advance and checked to be sure they are working properly. These should be arranged so that learners can see the demonstration; everyone must be able to see and hear easily. Use of assistants, mirrors, or television to increase the visibility and effectiveness of the demonstration may be considered. Rehearsing the demonstration and becoming familiar with the equipment is vital. Back-up equipment in case something fails is also essential. Student practice is basic and must be planned for. This is also a time-consuming process. A brief summarization on a handout will be helpful, especially when new equipment or procedures are being introduced.

After the above planning has occurred, the demonstration can be undertaken. The trainer's first consideration when presenting a demonstration is to let the learners know exactly what will be demonstrated. This introduction prepares the learners, sets a mood, and motivates the learners to pay close attention. Relating the lesson to previous and future knowledge sets a basis of understanding. Stating the objectives of the lesson lets learners know what they will have to perform after the demonstration. General health and safety rules should be stated at the beginning of the demonstration and repeated as needed. The instructor should state exactly what he is going to do before each step, explain what is happening and why the technique is used.

At the end of each major step, the instructor should check to be sure the technique is understood. The instructor must be sure to stand so that the learners are able to see and hear clearly. Learners should be alerted to a particularly difficult step. Each step should be summarized at the completion of the demonstration, and the learners' practice of the procedure supervised. Errors should be corrected immediately.

Demonstrations should follow the same format as lectures: introduction, body, and summary. They should also include practice, reinforcement, and learner evaluation. A good demonstration followed by adequate learner practice can often be more effective than can several lectures.

An inservice director should consider the method of presentation carefully. Using an inefficient presentation mode is functionless just as teaching without objectives is directionless.

Once the method of lecture or demonstration has been decided upon, the content must be prepared. Regardless of whether one chooses to present information in the lecture format or to demonstrate some new skill or technique, the first priority is to be both well informed and carefully prepared about the topic.

Preparing for lecturing and demonstration calls for making decisions about media in advance. Chapter 5 contains some pointers concerning media. Preparation also requires reviewing one's own motivation and the amount of time that can be devoted to preparation. It may be more efficient to utilize a more informed person on the nursing home's staff than to research a new topic. For example, the dietician might give a lecture on nutrition, or the activity director might give a demonstration on reality orientation methods. The training director can help the lecturer to plan the objectives, assist in locating media, resources, equipment, and can ensure that the presentation fits within the overall training goals.

Finally, an uncomfortable or uninformed audience will not be receptive to a speaker's message or demonstration. If possible, the trainer should prepare the learners by handing out appropriate materials. This allows the audience to be familiar with the lecture or demonstration topic before the program begins. Everyone in the audience must be able to see and hear the speaker; the room temperature must be kept at a comfortable level; a room appropriate to the number of people and the character of the lecture or demonstration must be chosen.

Group Discussions

Statistics tell us that more people lose their jobs because of an inability to get along with people than because of a lack of skill or knowledge. One solution to that problem is found in the small group discussion. This training technique helps people to become aware of each other. Trainers who employ this method are not only helping students to learn information, they are also helping students get along with each other and learn to work together. These skills will pay off immeasurably in the future. As society demands more people with human relations skills, trainers must take on the responsibility of helping learners to incorporate those skills into their working routines.

A small group discussion has the potential of being the most exciting teaching technique available. Students participate, share, and brainstorm to form decisions and opinions. The student becomes actively involved in the learning process, and the trainer moves from a position of dispenser of facts to facilitator of learning. This point is key in successful adult education.

Central to the small group is the concept of discussion, or group deliberation, focused on finding a cooperative solution to a problem or issue. Participants must be good listeners as well as speakers. No discussion is a one-way undertaking. The purpose of a small group discussion is to help clarify points of view while finding out what others think in order to reevaluate opinions. The trainer in this situation creates an atmosphere for self-directed learning. The role of center of attention is relinquished, and the trainer becomes an associate in the learning process. A good discussion topic interests the participants and suggests different points of view. The small group discussion technique is best used to encourage people to become aware of problems in the institution, to develop a nucleus of leadership, to identify and solve problems, and to decide on plans of action.

The advantages of using a small group discussion in training are many. Group discussion combines active participation and intellectual exercise and helps learners understand a topic with a clarity and vividness few other techniques can offer. Discussion also creates ideas while stimulating further study. Group members who feel a sense of community may be more inclined to assume responsibility for learning and for action on plans or activities formulated by the group. Working together to exchange ideas can result in friendship and acceptance. In addition, immediate feedback from others is acceptable in a group situation. Attitudes can, therefore, be openly discussed and, when appropriate, changed.

There are, however, some limitations to discussion as a training method. Only a limited number of participants can be involved if the discussion is to be effective. No more than twenty-five can effectively participate. If participants are not trained in discussion techniques, the group may be directionless. Some learners may not take responsibility for group learning, and not all topics lend themselves to discussion. A few people may dominate the discussion.

To a high degree, the success of a small group discussion

depends on the preparation put into it. Both trainer and learners must first understand their roles and the degree of participation required. Objectives must be concise and clear to all participants.

Because a discussion is basically an exchange of ideas, the room should physically encourage, rather than discourage, exchange. A circle or horseshoe arrangement is best. Face-to-face situations promote the exchange of ideas. Participants should be close enough to see and hear each other without straining. The optimum number of participants is from ten to twenty-five. More participants leads to chaos; fewer produces a lack of diversity and knowledge that is needed for an effective discussion.

In a small group discussion, the inservice director acts as a prompter, leading the learners to inferences and generalizations from the opinions presented. In *Freedom to Learn*, psychologist Carl Rogers addresses himself to the qualities that teachers should have: genuineness; acceptance of students as individuals; and empathic understanding of students (Rogers, 1969). These qualities are important in all teaching situations and are vital in discussions.

There are two tasks that the leader of discussions must accomplish: He must cover a certain amount of material, and he must involve students in discussion. Leaders who can create and maintain lively, factual, participative discussions are invaluable.

Standard ways to begin a discussion are to provide a common experience or problem, ask a question, or suggest a controversial opinion. Providing a concrete common experience may be done through a mutual reading assignment, a film, a demonstration, a lecture, or a role play. Problems can be presented by asking students to present a list they wish to talk about; this may be done as an assignment or during one of the initial discussion hours. The list begins an open exchange of ideas. Another method is to ask open-ended questions that have no correct answers but are not so abstract that they are puzzling or cannot be discussed. Also, a controversy or disagreement can begin a discussion. This can lead to learners voicing opposite opinions. The leader must, therefore, be ready to handle controversy within the group.

While it is easy to begin with questions, controversy, or common experience, the difficulty lies in maintaining the discussion. Trainers who can ask questions in a suggestive and meaningful fashion will find the discussions running more smoothly than those who have not mastered this questioning skill. There are several things a trainer can do to maintain the discussion. It is important to remember that smaller groups may handle a topic more easily than larger groups. Having facts on hand that relate to and clarify the topic can also help to direct arguments away from personal opinion. Asking learners to do some outside reading and to research topics is another way to center on factual information.

If the discussion begins to become unfocused, learners may write out their solution to the stated problem. Presenting these solutions to the group can refocus the discussion. The leader may also form "buzz groups" to air the topic. After a designated time, the groups share their findings with the total group. Calling on people directly, asking open-ended question, and providing more information when necessary are further ways to bring the discussion into focus. The conflict should be focused on ideas rather than on personalities. Learners should be encouraged to talk directly to each other instead of through the instructor. Feelings and opinions should be encouraged before moving to fact. At times, it is more productive to respond to feelings rather than to the content of a statement.

A small group will not be effective unless the trainer uses certain skills, attitudes, and knowledge in leading the students to the planned objectives. However, the trainer will have to give up his role as center of attention, as well as the misconception that he is not working unless he is talking. Listening and responding techniques are critical. Silence, while often a sign of boredom or confusion, can signify thought. Therefore, a trainer must be sensitive to the progress of the session, and must avoid taking a heavy hand when it is not called for.

In summary, the discussion is an excellent method of involving adults in learning. It is an active, rather than passive, mode of learning. Feedback is immediate. Participant feedback can allow the trainer to focus and evaluate during the presentation and to adjust and amend the discussion as needed.

Use of Lecture, Demonstration, and Discussion: Examples

Suppose you are preparing the material involved in teaching aides to take vital signs. Looking at the objectives for vital signs presented in Chapter 3, one can see that some of these will be better accomplished by use of the lecture, whereas others require demonstration, and another may be accomplished best via discussion. The examples below take the objectives in the order in which they were presented.

Objective 1.   By the end of this inservice training, aides will be able to demonstrate the correct method of taking oral temperature. It becomes quickly obvious that a demonstration is inappropriate; it would suffer the limitation of all students not being able to see the instructor's view of the thermometer, both before and after demonstrating the procedure. In addition, students would never be able to see the markings and mercury. It is obvious that a discussion would suffer from the limitation pertaining to the nature of the topic: There is a prescribed method for taking and reading oral temperatures, and nothing would be gained by stimulating a discussion about it. Therefore, the lecture method is the best possibility. It has the advantage of allowing the information to be presented quickly to a large number of people, and visual aids can be easily incorporated. Since a single thermometer is too difficult for a group to see, a large-scale drawing may be useful during the explanation.

Objective 2.   By the end of this inservice training, aides will be able to write three valid reasons for using a rectal thermometer instead of an oral thermometer. Small group discussions may be appropriate for attaining this objective. Although the same reasoning applies to this as to the previous objective in most respects, one further factor must be considered. The oral technique of taking vital signs has already been taught; the rectal technique is very similar. Therefore, the educational intent involves differentiating between conditions requiring the use of one method over the other. A good discussion may bring out good ideas about when to use each method, and the instructor can allow students to exchange examples and draw their own conclusions. Any situations not covered by the group can be supplied by the instructor.

Objective 3.   After watching a demonstration on how to take the pulse rate, aides will be able to write instructions for this procedure. The decision for this objective is easy since the use of demonstration is already involved. A lecture method could actually be used, but is is wise to vary teaching methodology, and lecturing tends to predominate over other techniques. This objective lends itself as well or better than do the others to the use of demonstration since all students can see (and copy) the instructor. The use of discussion is probably not appropriate for the same reason that it was rejected with Objective 1.

Objective 4. After three trials, the aide will be able to demonstrate taking another person's blood pressure, correctly describing the process involved. In this case the decision of teaching method is less clear cut. While small group discussion may be inappropriate for learning this standard procedure, either a lecture or demonstration could be used. In fact, one could incorporate the advantages of both teaching methods by giving a combined lecture-demonstration. Since taking blood pressure is somewhat more complicated than taking temperature or pulse, presenting the information orally through a lecture and visually through a demonstration will enhance learning.

Objective 5.   Given a sample of vital signs, the aide will be able to record the information in proper form in the TPR notebook. As noted earlier, when something the size of a TPR notebook must be seen by a group, it is probably best not to use the demonstration technique. When a standard procedure is being explained, the use of a small group discussion is probably inappropriate. However, a lecture using an enlarged representation of the notebook should pose no learning or teaching problems.

This example presents some of the points that should be considered when choosing the presentation mode. The methods presented in subsequent chapters should also be considered. It is important to remember that the method of presentation ensure that the instructional objectives are met in the most efficient and effective manner.

Chapter 5
Media

Using Media Effectively

Very often, trainers consider using media too late. Other training considerations occupy their minds and anything that supplements the basic lecture or demonstration seems a frill. In other cases, the trainer may think of taking slides or of drawing a chart, but with the lecture scheduled for the next day, there is no time to prepare media that will have impact.

The time to begin developing audiovisual aides is during the preliminary outlining of the training course. A trainer should ask: "What are the primary ideas that I want to get across to my audience?" and "Are there effective ways of presenting these ideas other than by words?"

Explaining a concept through the medium of words is an exercise in abstraction; that is, each member of the audience will create his own mental image of what is being said. Speakers can only hope that their words are creating the correct impression. A slide or a picture dramatizes a concept, placing the words in a more concrete form. Research has shown that people remember only 10 percent of what they read, 20 percent of what they hear, and 30 percent of what they see. Learning in several receiving modes increases retention: Seeing and hearing in combination increase retention to 50 percent; and explaining to others while using visual aids increases retention to 90 percent (Dale, 1954).

Before trainers begin the process of selecting instructional media for their programs, however, they must have a firm grasp of the objectives of the lesson. Once an objective is defined in behavioral terms, the selection of media should mesh with the lesson plan to form an effective program.

There are many reasons for using thoughtfully prepared media, both in the area of technical competence and in educational content. They provide sensory stimuli by allowing learners to look at or listen to something other than the speaker. However, because the novelty wears off rapidly, unless the media are of high quality, training aids will lose their interest. Media clarify concepts by showing relationships, outlining the progression of ideas, or illustrating applications. Media can initiate a discussion more quickly than can a speaker. Sometimes individuals are reluctant to begin discussing certain subjects or perhaps they don't know where to begin; a short film, by dramatizing one aspect of the subject, can provoke spontaneous comments, and a skillful teacher can lead the audience from this starting point. With some modification, media can be adapted for the purpose of self-study and review. By using the same materials included in a lecture, a trainer can design a short refresher course that will recall the ideas the audience should remember. Media are, however, only as good as the person who uses them. Effective use of media will depend on a knowledge of the basic principles underlying their use.

Visual media are used in addition to words and gestures in order to help get the message across. They are supplements and reinforcements to the content presented by the trainer. A visual could be used (American Hospital Association, 1978):

- to make a point that is too complex or abstract for spoken words alone
- to clarify a point that evokes different mental images between learners
- when all learners need to see the same thing
- when a high level of retention is desired
- to hold or gain attention
- to summarize points.

Nonprojected Media

Visual or nonprojected media that can be used in inservice programs are: drawings and illustrations; models or mock-ups; chalk board; flip charts; simulators; real objects; and independent study units.

Nonprojected material should be kept simple and should ilustrate only one major idea. They should be large enough for all learners to see easily; they are most useful when displayed or mounted. If visual materials, models, or real objects are available to learners for careful viewing after the inservice, they act as additional reinforcement.

Drawings and Illustrations

Drawings and illustrations can include posters, graphs, charts, and line drawings. Two special types of drawings that are particularly useful for inservice directors are cartoons and handouts. Drawings can range from highly simplified, trainer-produced drawings to those that are commercially produced in full color. They can be used alone or as part of a display.

Often they are converted to slides or overhead transparencies and are used to emphasize primary points in lectures and demonstrations. Drawings and illustrations have the advantage of being easily located, inexpensive, and suited for independent or small groups. Good illustrations attract attention, arouse interest, clarify meanings, and simplify complex information.

Cartoons

Cartoons used in the nursing home setting can stimulate and encourage staff to examine current practices, behavior, values, and expectations; they may help staff to consider and implement changes to make treatment more therapeutic and life more meaningful for the elderly. Posters offer an excellent way for a trainer to utilize a cartoon. Commercial cartoons that are appropriate commentary can be posted along with thought-provoking questions. For example, Cartoons 1, 2,

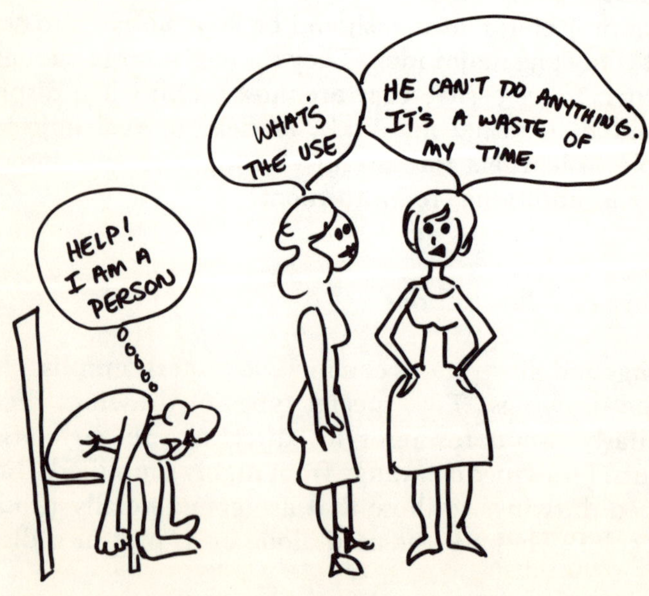

Cartoon 1

and 3 portray some common staff attitudes in nursing homes. Questions considering such issues as sexuality among the aged, staff-resident communication, and patient rights could all be used. Inservice participants could also be asked to draw their own cartoons. This is particularly useful for initiating discussion on controversial topics or staff problems. For example, one staff member may draw a cartoon like Cartoon 4, which portrays administrative attitudes.

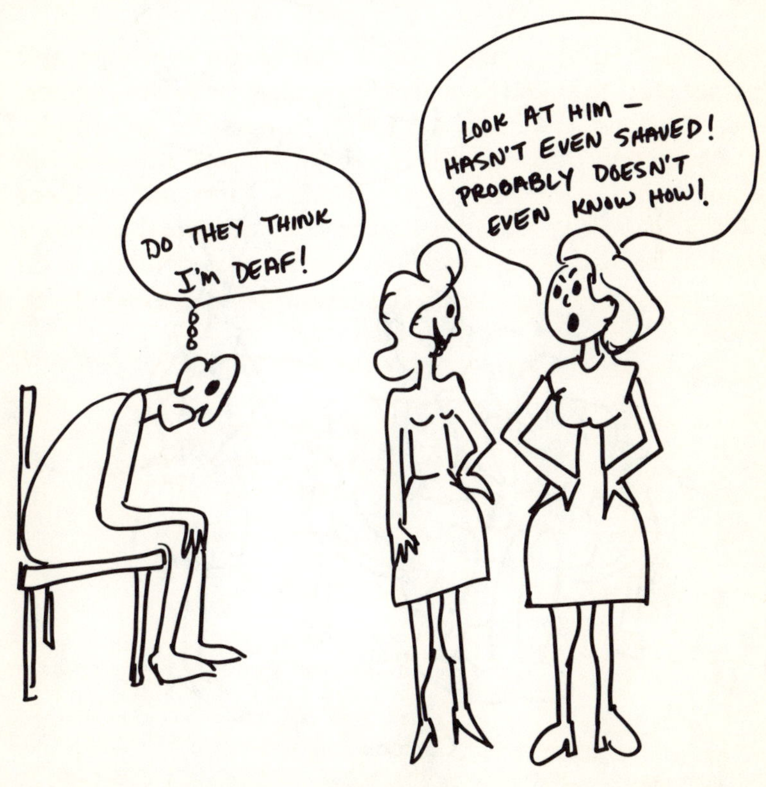

Cartoon 2

The exercise of creating a cartoon that concerns the participants' own setting is a technique that could facilitate discussion about negative attitudes and practices in a non-threatening way. The cartoons may focus on issues relating to nontherapeutic practices in such areas as staff relationships, administrative practices, and staff communication with residents.

Using humor in the learning environment can prove to be a valuable technique for eliciting feelings and attitudes toward a variety of issues in the long-term care setting. It can add variety to the various teaching methods.

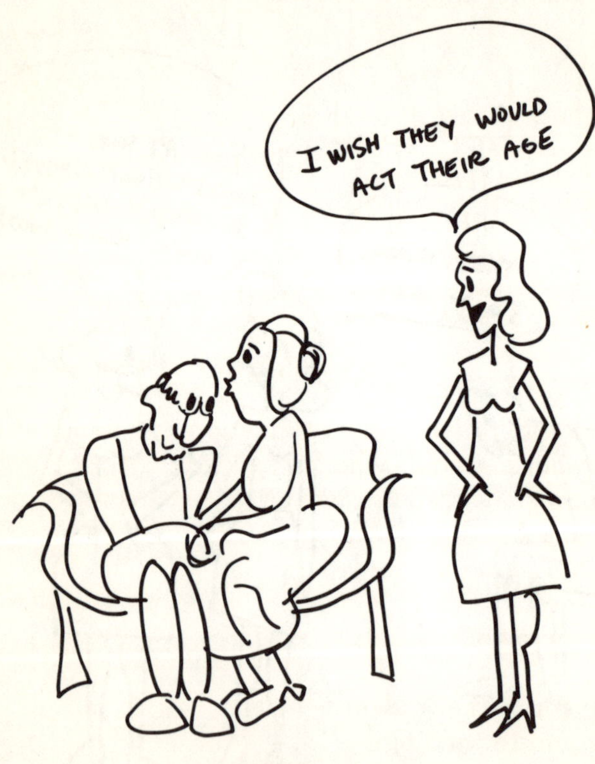

Cartoon 3

Handouts

Most trainers agree that handouts are an important method of reinforcing teaching. They can clearly organize and standardize all the necessary information that is given to staff members.

ADMINISTRATIVE POLICY

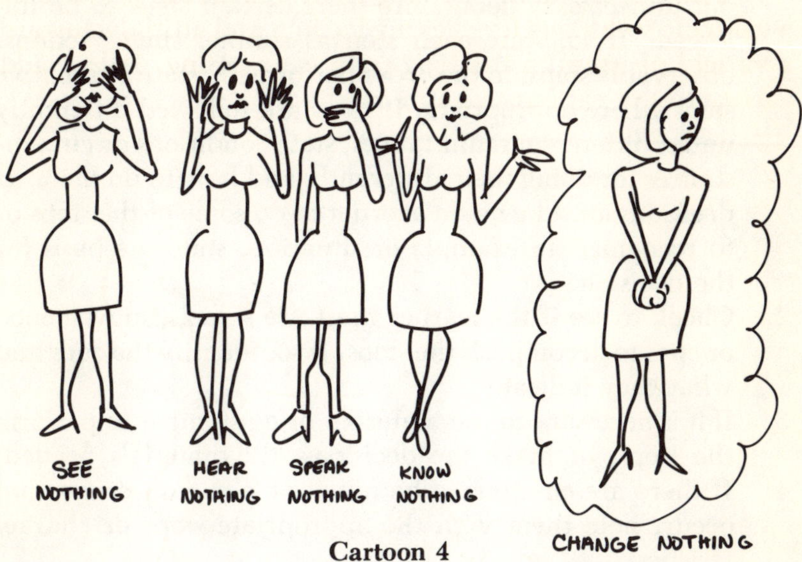

Cartoon 4

Careful consideration to the production of a handout is essential. Handout material, whether quizzes, outlines, lists, or reprinted newspaper articles, can either be effective or wasteful. Too often a handout ends up in the wastebasket. Trainers should plan handouts to suit the lesson's objectives and the learners' needs. Before making a handout consider that a handout must be:

- pertinent to the student
- short and to the point
- immediately and obviously valuable to the student
- stimulating and involving
- legible, or no one will read it no matter how good its information

Before preparing a handout, the following steps should be taken:

1. Decide what the objective requires the learner to do. Do you need to state facts? If so, state them simply and without unnecessary detail. Are there certain steps to be followed? If so, state each step as simple, single actions, observable steps, in the order performed; state alternative steps where appropriate. If steps are followed differently under different circumstances, state conditions or circumstances for doing them differently and how to do them. If decisions must be made in order to do some of the steps or to recognize an example or situation, state the basis for the decision.
2. Check to see if the learner must use signals, movements, or cues to accomplish the steps. If so, identify the cues and what they indicate.
3. If it is necessary to use materials or equipment to perform the steps, or make the decisions, list materials needed.
4. If there are cautions to be noted or common errors that occur, note them with the appropriate steps or characteristics.
5. If possible, provide a simple rationale for learning the facts, steps, or decisions.
6. Check the information to ensure that it excludes nonessential technical vocabulary or explains it, and that it contains complete and accurate information (Freedman, 1978).

Once the basic information to be included has been determined, the handout itself should include: a title, a description of when the information on the handout should be used and the materials necessary; a list of needed information; labels for the examples; highlights of common errors and cautions. If drawings are used, label diagrams or illustrations in order to make the meaning clear, eliminate unneeded detail, and clarify the context. Use a variety of techniques to create interest: type size, style, boldness for titles and key points; color for emphasis and colored sheets for easy identification; arrows, circled or enlarged sections to point out areas of interest; boxes, double lines, asterisks, or symbols to set aside key information; double columns for commenting on information in the text.

An important consideration for many nursing home staff is reading level. Materials developed must be on a comprehensible level. One way to check a handout for reading level is by performing a readability test. There are many formulas for this; most use vocabulary, word length, sentence length or number of ideas in a paragraph as an index of reading difficulty. The Fog Index developed by Robert Gunning (1968) is one method. To calculate the Fog Index of any written material, a hundred-word sample of the material is taken. The average length of sentence in that sample is then found by counting the number of sentences, stopping at the period nearest the hundred-word mark. Next, the number of sentences is divided into the number of words contained in the sentences, after which the percentage of hard words contained in the number of words in those sentences is found. This is done by counting the words with three or more syllables and dividing that number by the total number of words. A word whose third syllable is the suffix "-ed" or "-es," as in the word "sentences," should be included. Hyphenated or compound words that merely combine easy words, as in "hundred-word," are not included. Finally, to obtain the Fog Index, the average sentence length and the percentage of hard words are added, then multiplied by 0.4. The answer is the school grade level necessary to easily read the passage.

A sample calculation of the language used in these instructions explaining the Fog Index can be done by first counting 100 words beginning at "The Fog Index developed by . . ." in the preceding paragraph. The hundreth word is "and" in the sentence beginning "This is done by counting . . ." The period that follows the word is closer than the period that precedes it. Therefore, the Fog Index for this passage will be based on the first five sentences. These sentences contain 109 words. The average length of sentence is 109 divided by 5, or 21.8. Sixteen words of three or more syllables are contained in the five sentences that end with "the total number of words." These words are: developed, calculate, material (twice), average, sentences (4 times), period, divided, percentage, syllables, and dividing. The percentage of hard words is 14 divided by 109, or .129 or 13 percent. The Fog Index is 21.8 +13 = 34.8 x 0.4 = 13.9. This means that this sample of material is on a college reading level and is of too difficult a level for inservice handouts. A low Fog Index of 5.0 to 6.0 is recommended for staff handouts.

Once the handout has been checked to make sure that it is clear, concise, and readable, it should be tested; that is, it may be used in training while stopping for questions or problems. Observations concerning how the handout is used in training and whether or not it is kept by trainees and used later in the facility, may prove useful. If the handout was successful it should be kept for future use. If not, it can be discarded.

Using the vital signs objectives again, a sample of a handout concerning reading thermometers is shown in Figure 5.1. The various parts of the handout are marked.

Handouts are useful teaching tools if they are pertinent, short, legible, and motivational. They can provide an excellent transfer aid. By giving the learner a step-by-step list of ways to apply his newly acquired concepts and skills, the trainer gives the learner a schedule for application. In this manner, the desired instructional outcomes are reinforced for efficient use.

Models, Mock-ups, Simulators, Objects

Models, mock-ups, simulators, and real objects are other types of nonprojected media often used in inservice. Models and mock-ups are three-dimensional representations of objects

TAKING A TEMPERATURE WITH A GLASS THERMOMETER

Materials needed

TPR book
Thermometer in a container
  of sterilizing solution
Tissues
Wristwatch with a second
  hand
Lubricant (if using rectal
  thermometer)

Procedure

Remove thermometer from its container
Wipe thermometer with tissue
Check the reading; shake and recheck
  until reading is below 96
Insert thermometer, noticing time
Count pulse and respirations
Remove thermometer after
  3 minutes' time
Wipe thermometer with tissue
Read and record temperature in TPR
  book
Shake down thermometer; return it to
  its container

CAUTION: You will find it necessary to shake the thermometer vigorously in order to get a reading below 96. Be sure that your arm has enough room so that you avoid personal injury and the hazard of broken glass.

Example

Both the rectal and oral thermometers below have readings below 96.

Rectal Thermometer

Oral Thermometer

Where would the mercury stand if the reading was normal? Practice drawing in the mercury on these thermometers:

Rectal Thermometer

Oral Thermometer

NOTE: Aged people often have difficulty regulating body temperature. Therefore, you may consider a reading as low as 97 by mouth and 98 by rectum to be normal temperatures for geriatric patients.

Figure 5.1.   Sample Handout

that differ from the real object in size, material, and/or function. Mock-ups differ from models in their usually larger size and their moving and operating parts. An example of a mock-up is a replica of the circulatory system in which a red liquid is pumped through clear plastic tubing.

Simulators are apparatuses used in the teaching of a skill or procedure. They are mock-up devices for skill practice. Equipment simulators are used to teach such things as self-injection of drugs or mouth-to-mouth resuscitation by using simulators of a rubber arm or head and lung.

Real objects are commonly used in inservice when staff is expected to learn how to manipulate a particular object or to be able to work equipment. Real objects should be integrated into a total demonstration. Adequate time should be included for practice and feedback.

Independent Study Units

Independent study units are an under-utilized medium in inservice. They can, however, be quite effective with one or two learners or in cases such as orientation, when the content may be continuously repeated. Independent study units can be as simple as a page of written instructions or a short procedure manual or more complex forms, including slide-sound presentations, filmstrips, videotapes, or computer assisted instruction. They can be individual trainer prepared or commercially produced. They should contain all the information and concepts that the learner will need to attain the learning objectives. Before learners begin, necessary background information should be supplied, independent of group instruction. The trainer should start the learner through the unit by discussing the objectives and explaining any instructions. Sufficient time to answer questions and to practice demonstrated skills, as well as to visualize key concepts is needed. An independent study unit may end with the trainer's initiating a follow-up session to clarify concepts and to reinforce learning.

The following suggestions will guide the trainer to a professional use of nonprojected media, so that ideas may be simply presented and implemented without overcomplicated visuals.

1. Decide which ideas merit emphasis; that is, which concepts are difficult to grasp if not visualized.
2. Carefully limit the number of objectives for each presentation. Keep things simple and to the point.
3. For each segment of instruction determine appropriate content and media format of the material to be used.
4. Announce the purpose of the media materials to the learners. Materials are most effective when they provoke interest, anticipation, and readiness to respond (Allen & Seifman, 1971).

Other considerations to remember when selecting media are the cost implications (that is, production, replacement, rental charges, energy); time available to secure and show materials; and size of the audience. Projected media, including programmed materials, audio recordings, photographic slides, overhead transparencies, filmstrips, videotapes, and motion pictures, are commonly used in training programs. Major considerations in considering use of projected media are locating resources and equipment. Many local and university libraries, pharmaceutical companies, and film associations have projected media for loan or rent. Judicious telephoning can usually result in a number of media catalogues. In addition, several university gerontology centers have regional film collections on topics pertinent to nursing home staff. These are listed in the resource list at the end of this chapter.

Decisions about equipment usually depend on the trainer's choice of materials; sometimes the type of equipment available may influence the form of the material to be used. For example, although slides might be preferred, if filmstrip viewers are available, are much less expensive, and are easier to use than slide projectors, the trainer may decide to use filmstrips. Careful consideration to availability and usability of equipment during planning is essential. Before requesting equipment, the trainers must think in terms of available funds, the complexity of the equipment, and upkeep expenses.

Most people have had experience using audiovisual and related resources. However, knowledge and judgment concerning the advantages, limitations, and special applications of these materials are limited. The following list of questions is provided as a guide for evaluating and selecting these materials:

1. Do the materials contribute meaningful cognitive or affective content to the topic under study? Does the medium appear to be one that will complement and advance the instructional objectives, or will it simply fill classroom time?
2. Does the medium give a clear picture of the ideas it was designed to present? Are there distortions in the content such as incorrect facts, inadequate sampling or representations, or obsolescence? If the medium expresses distortions yet offers valuable content, the instructor should mention inaccuracies prior to the presentation.
3. Can the audiovisual materials aid students in developing critical thinking capabilities? Some audiovisuals have a persuasive charm; others stimulate analytical and logical thought. Where these consequences are desired, does the medium lull viewers into passive acceptance when critical examination and judgment are needed? How and to what extent does the medium promote critical thinking?
4. Is the material appropriate to the age, intelligence, and experience levels of the learners? To enhance learning of

individuals new to the field of gerontology, students should be able to relate some of the medium's content to individual or shared life experiences. Unrelated, unintegrated content can be readily lost or forgotten by the learner.

5. Is the technical or physical quality of the materials satisfactory? Sometimes a medium's content is of sufficient value that faulty or poor technical quality can render a message virtually useless.

6. Is the material worth the time, expense, and effort involved? Is a film, record or picture more valuable than some other experience in meeting instructional objectives? What is the relative value of a film or videotape to the teaching program when equipment rental costs are considered? Are the media valuable enough to justify the time and effort of the instructor?

7. Is there a teacher's guide to effective use of the media? Not all media require an instructor's guide. When available, guides and handbooks are often useful. However, some guides are developed without prior experimentation with the media, while others offer general suggestions that are not specifically applicable to a particular course or instructional unit.

After commercial media material is located, it should be previewed and evaluated. The evaluation should include the title, the medium, the source, the program source, and the cost. The medium should also be viewed in the context of how well it meets the learning objectives and how it will be used in presentation. It is helpful to file this information, as well as general impressions concerning technical aspects, for future reference. Grading the material can also aid future selection.

When using someone else's movies, videotapes, or slide tapes for a presentation, the following precautions should be observed:

1. Preview the material beforehand and make sure that only materials that relate to the objectives and the needs of the learners are used.
2. Restate the objective and the points of particular interest before showing the material.
3. Use only what meets your needs if the entire program is not appropriate.
4. Point out any terms or steps that are different from the ones already used.
5. At the start of the presentation, check to make sure each viewer can see and hear adequately.
6. At the end of the presentation, key points should be summarized or questions covering the points asked.
7. If the presentation teaches the staff to do something, they should try to perform it immediately after summary or questions. The chance to review the materials before practice should be offered.
8. If props, equipment, or materials are needed to perform the objective, they should be ready.

Projected visuals are valuable in that they attract and hold attention; at the same time, they have the ability to show great detail to several people at once. Disadvantages primarily involve the equipment technicalities and logistics.

Summary

Reviewing the original objectives for teaching aides how to read vital signs can help to summarize selecting the correct medium for use in the inservice. Considering each of the five objectives individually, the following selections become clear.

Objective 1.   Since a single thermometer is too small for a group, a large-scale representation will be needed. This could be a large drawing on poster paper, an overhead transparency, or individual handouts. These would probably show the thermometer at several different readings.

Objective 2.   A drawing of a rectal thermometer with the visual aide for Objective 1 could easily be included. Following the discussion, a trainer might list on a flip chart the reasons the group found for using one temperature-taking technique in place of the other.

Objective 3.   It might be worthwhile to videotape a demonstration of the pulse-taking procedure. This would allow dubbing an audio signal to represent the pulse. In addition, the trainer then has the flexibility to stop and repeat the film if desired.

Objective 4.   Since this objective may be met with a combined teaching technique, media may be selected for each. During the lecture phase, actual equipment, large pictures, transparencies, or handouts may be used. During the demonstration the actual equipment will most certainly be needed. Of course it may be included in a videotape, should you make one for the other demonstrations. Taking vital signs is such a common procedure, and one that is so often used, there may be existing films, filmstrips, or slide tape presentations which cover this information.

Objective 5.   The lecture method for this objective has been identified. An enlarged replication of a page from the TPR notebook will probably facilitate teaching. You may also want to make a handout of a sample blank page for students to use for practice.

Audiovisual Sources

American Nursing Home Association, Film Service, Box 7316, Alexandria, VA 22307

Concept Media, 1500 Adams Avenue, Costa Mesa, CA 92626

Gerontology Film Collection, Main Library, North Texas State University, Denton, TX 76203

Roche Laboratories, Division of Hoffman-LaRoche Industries, Nutley, NJ 07110

Sandoz Pharmaceuticals, Division of Sandoz-Wander, 59 State Highway #10, Hanover, NJ 07936

United Hospital Fund, 3 East 54th Street, New York, NY 10022

University of Michigan, Audiovisual Education Center, 416 Fourth Street, Ann Arbor, MI 48104

University of Southern California, Division of Cinema—Film Distribution Center, University Park, Los Angeles, CA 90007

Wayne State University, Audio Visual Productions Center, 680 Putnam, Detroit, MI 48202

Film Catalogs

About Aging: A Catalog of Films: Andrus Gerontology Center, University of Southern California, Los Angeles, CA 90007

Media/Resources for Gerontology: Institute of Gerontology, University of Michigan, Ann Arbor, MI 48104

Film Catalog—Publication No. 5218: American Hospital Association, 860 North Lake Shore Drive, Chicago, IL 60611

Film Catalog—Management: Film Department, American Management Association, 135 West 50th Street, New York, NY 10020

Gerontological Film Collection Catalog: Gerontological Film Collection, Main Library, North Texas State University, Denton, TX 76203

Chapter 6
Situational Learning

Along with the teaching of techniques of lecture, demonstration, and discussion, several other methods of presenting material to adult students are available to perceptive trainers. These methods include case study, role playing, and simulation games. Each can be viewed independently, or combined with another method. For example, a role play can be easily followed by a discussion, or a case study can grow out of a role play. The following brief discussions of each of these methods should help trainers to understand when they can best be used.

Case Method

In the case study method of teaching, learners use a factual history or description of an event as a springboard for learning how to deal with a particular situation. The case may be real or fictitious. It is put together to present a principle the trainer wants to convey. The cases, which always involve group discussion, expose a part of organizational life to the learners without providing clear-cut answers.

There are several advantages to using a case study method approach. One major advantage is that learners actively participate by expressing their own views and opinions. They learn from each other as well as from the trainer. They gain practice in thinking of themselves and others in various roles within the nursing home. Sessions are interesting mixes of participation and dialogue. Adults tend to like this method since the realistic cases are intrinsically interesting and relate directly to current job experiences.

There are some limitations, however, to the case study method approach. Learners not used to this method may initially feel frustrated by the lack of direction, and they may think they are wasting their time. Some content areas cannot be easily taught through a series of cases. Progress in development of problem solving and administrative skills may be slow. Usually a case study assumes a basic knowledge of the facts as well as certain skills, maturity, and readiness to accept responsibility. Case studies may emphasize positive decisions when negative decisions are the best action. Cases tend to simplify real world situations, in part because inclusion of all the variables actually involved would be too long or cumbersome.

While preparing for a case study, a trainer should study it carefully, making sure the case is suitable for the objectives and for the level of learner. The trainer must imagine the way in which the learner will read the material. Will the learner comprehend the subtleties of the case? Will he focus on words that have different meanings than those the trainer had in mind? Sometimes trainers unfairly label learners as slow or dense when the fault is their own because of the way training materials were constructed.

At the time the case is first introduced, the trainer makes clear, through the lecture method, what objectives are to be achieved. The discussion that follows the study should emphasize that the goal of case study is attainment of a better system of problem solving as opposed to a secure answer to one isolated problem.

In presenting the case materials, the material should be written for all the participants and read aloud to allow for verbal emphasis of certain points. As participants discuss the case, the trainer must be alert for learners who get off the track, those who misinterpret the case, or those who discuss unrelated topics. The room's atmosphere is important. As in a small group, a circle or horseshoe arrangement of chairs best encourages interaction. The group should be limited to twenty participants. All participants should be able to see and hear comfortably. At the end of the discussion, the trainer should summarize the case and the conclusions. This is also the time to point out alternative solutions, similar cases, or other important information.

While case studies are available on topics as wide-ranging as motivation of staff members to dealing with complaints, the most effective study will be that which specifically relates to the participants and their environment. Published case materials may save time for a trainer, but they should not be used if they do not fit the objectives and level of the group. Trainees must be able to visualize the link between themselves and the case, or the effort is wasted. The case materials developed within a particular nursing home can be effective in practically all areas of inservice training, including discipline, communications, grievances, morale, and productivity. In evaluating and preparing case materials, the trainer must consider language, content, and length of the study.

The language must convey what the trainer intends it to convey. Words should be the simplest needed to explain ideas and transmit the exact message and meaning. Sentences need to be short and clear. Technical expressions should be easily understood or defined. Ideas and concepts should be presented in logical order. In addition, learners in nursing home settings may often have low levels of reading ability; too often learners are labeled slow or uncooperative when, in reality, the material presented is not on an appropriate reading level.

The content must be appropriate in both level and topic. The complexity of the materials should be suitable for the group. It cannot be so simple that it is not interesting, nor can it be insulting to the level of the learner. All essential material must be presented. Extraneous materials having no relevance to the facts or to setting the scene should be avoided, as should case situations in which learners were involved. All essential material should be presented.

Mood, tone, or humor can be used to elicit desired outcomes. Emotionalism should be avoided. The case situation should be one with which the group can readily identify. Use of realistic situations within nursing home settings is excellent.

The length of the case must fit the training time. The cases cannot be too complete, or little is left for learners to discuss. If the case is incomplete, the group may flounder and not proceed in the desired direction. The length of the case needs to be suitable for the time available for discussion, as discussion is vital with the case study approach.

Whatever the particular objectives for a training session, the trainer should write the case study focusing on those objectives. The case itself will be a significant factor in reaching those objectives. A poorly constructed case will only hamper a trainer's efforts.

The two widely used techniques of case writing are inductive and deductive. Inductive cases are those that tell about given situations and lead to a conclusion or a basic principle. Deductive cases begin with the principle and and then present situations and examples. In other words, the case may be presented from either the top down or from the bottom up.

In writing an inductive case, the trainer should choose

familiar situations from the work environment. The case should be job-related and have intrinsic value as a potential learning exercise. The next step is to evaluate or judge the situation by analyzing the available facts and inferences. Next, the problem and its related principle should be decided upon. Then, if feasible, the situation's resolution should be found. Since many problems are never completely solved or are solved erroneously, this factor is not essential to case construction. The final step is to establish a fictionalized version of the original situation, changing the names, titles, places, and times.

In writing a deductive case, the trainer selects a general principle to be illustrated as an instructional objective. For example, the trainer may choose to illustrate that supervisors have a training responsibility in orienting new employees. This principle is clarified and elaborated on within the written case. The case study may explain what occurs in a job situation if the defined principle is not applied by a supervisor. The case establishes a problem situation that includes as many of the situational factors as can be realistically fictionalized. The case should appear in a format that includes a warm-up introduction with key background data, the real or fictional problem, and the predicament. The case should end with questions or an assignment directed at the learner. The final questions challenge the group while channeling energies to the intended goal.

Both inductive and deductive cases can be used in training. By using cases, the trainer can present realistic situations. This involves learners in learning and motivates interest in the learning activities.

Following is an example of a case study that might be used in a nursing home. Consider again the objectives concerning vital signs that were used as examples in the preceding chapters. Perhaps the educational intent of the inservice extends beyond teaching basic techniques for obtaining vital signs. A situation in which aides are able to perform these procedures adequately when tested, but encounter difficulties in the actual work setting, may occur. Many activities are occurring simultaneously on the floor, and patient care is often complicated by these interacting conditions. Therefore, the inservice objectives include some general principles of patient care related to the taking of vital signs. As mentioned, the case study offers an excellent opportunity to do this.

Sample Case Study

Mrs. Bad Temper, a patient on your floor, has just had an altercation with a volunteer who brought her a requested cup of hot coffee. Mrs. Bad Temper drank the coffee, insisted it was poisoned by the volunteer, then used the empty cup to strike the volunteer. The charge nurse was alerted and received the same treatment while trying to disarm the patient. This was not the first time Mrs. Bad Temper had attacked others. Since her attacks are usually followed by throwing all loose objects at passersby, placing her arms in restraint has been the only viable solution to this problem. It seems that Mrs. Bad Temper becomes highly aggressive in conjunction with her history of fecal impactions. Meanwhile, her food tray is arriving and you are scheduled to take her vital signs. What should you do?

Following the procedures outlined for a case study, the inservice director would present the objectives, give a copy of the narrative to each student, and read it aloud. Participants would then be invited to discuss the situation. The inservice director would circulate in order to clarify and keep the discussion focused on the topic. Following the discussion, the participants would be asked for some examples of what aides would do in the situation. This opportunity can be used to point out several principles of patient care. These may include:

1. When in doubt about proceeding with an assignment, check with the charge nurse.
2. Oral temperature is never taken immediately after a patient has consumed a hot beverage.
3. If the arms are restrained, respiration rate cannot be checked by observing the arm on the chest or the pulse at the wrist. Alternative procedures must be used.
4. When the anus is irritated, rectal temperature should not be taken.
5. Oral temperature is never taken when the patient is confused or highly agitated.
6. Keep the patient's best interest in mind when deciding how important it is to proceed with an assignment.
7. Try to remain calm in disturbing situations since anxiety will only add more tension.

These principles are not intended to be exhaustive, but rather illustrative of the kinds of information one can convey through use of the case study. Some specific policies and procedures observed by your individual institution can also be identified. These might include:

- the procedure for serving a late meal
- how to note the necessity for skipping some or all of the vital signs procedure
- incident report procedure
- restraint policy

At the conclusion of the case study presentation, the in-service director should summarize the main points of the discussion (that is, those that reflect the objectives) which were brought out in the case study.

Role Playing

Role playing, the acting out of a situation by members of a learning group, is an active learning experience. Through role playing, learners simulate relationships and problems in advance, so they can anticipate appropriate behavior in on-the-job situations. After the role playing learners often move into small groups to discuss the action and agree on the most appropriate course.

In the role playing a person temporarily adopts a specified role and tries to behave in ways characteristic of a person in that role. For example, in a role play scene illustrating the need for staff-patient communication, one learner will play an overworked nurse and another will play a demanding patient. Given a particular set of circumstances and a setting, the two strive to resolve the problem by acting out the situation.

Role playing offers a chance to try out attitudes and behaviors that might be otherwise inappropriate or unavailable. Playing roles opposite to one's usual role (for example, client instead of worker) helps staff to develop empathy with that opposing role and helps to improve professional performance. Role playing is usually thought to be fun for the students. It is often more effective than the instructor's merely telling the students how to act. Role playing often provides good feedback for the instructor.

The trainer should consider several points before choosing role play as a teaching method. Role playing depends heavily on imagination and capacity to project into another situation. Role playing can be time consuming, especially if repeated many times, with staff playing a variety of roles. The technique is not easy to use effectively and some groups may be afraid of it.

In preparing for the role playing situation the trainer must define the objectives for the role play situation, study the background of the participants, determine the problem and situation to be portrayed, and determine the roles to be played. The leader will also determine if a particular scene needs to be played twice. For example, the trainer may wish to show both an effective and ineffective way for a staff member to deal with a demanding patient through role play.

The role play is never rehearsed. The leader briefs the participants as to their parts. The briefing can be either verbal or it can include a written description. Objectives and characters are explained. Behaviors are not. The leader also prepares an introduction for the group that helps them to understand the objectives and characterizations they will see.

The leader is an essential element in the effective use of role play. It is the leader's job to set the stage and to help the learners initiate the situation. Learners often become nervous or afraid when asked to participate. These feelings can be alleviated by fostering an open, supportive attitude and by helping participants begin. One way to do this is to have the trainer participate in one of the first role plays.

Once the situation has been carefully planned by the trainer, the role play itself involves many things. Spontaneity is a hallmark of effective role playing. The participants improvise their script as they speak, and the make-believe situation is acted upon by the participants as if it were real. The enactment must be as sincere and realistic as possible. This is neither a game nor a charade. The participants are interacting as if they were alone, without others listening and observing the action. Any attempts by participants to ham it up and show brilliant repartee and witticism should be avoided. Deliberately confusing and confounding the facts by inserting erroneous or misleading information into the role should also be discouraged.

The trainer sets the tone for the role play by clearly delineating the ground rules and boundaries while directing the action. The trainer is free to stop the action at any time. At the end of the role play the trainer should summarize the learning activity. Group discussion concerning the manner in which the participants interacted can be used to aid learning and to summarize points.

An example of a role play using the same material presented in the case study follows.

Sample Role Play

Perhaps the objectives of the inservice are not so much concerned with the learners knowing the principles, policies, and procedures outlined above, but are more concerned with professional behavior. Therefore, the case study situation can be narrated and the roles of Mrs. Bad Temper, the nurses' aide, and the volunteer can be assigned to be played by various learners. They are then asked to act out the scene as if it were actually happening. This provides a graphic demonstration of the complexity of interaction which can occur. At the close of the role playing scene, the group can discuss and evaluate the most appropriate responses, offering additional options for handling the situation. Some outcomes might be the following:

1. Aides develop greater empathy for the patient, the volunteer, and dietary staff.
2. Aides become sensitized to handling sticky situations in a professional manner.
3. The inservice director obtains good feedback in areas in which more training is needed, in which potential problems exist, and in which skill levels are high.

Simulation Games

Games usually involve a simulation of real world situations and processes, often in a simplified or dramatic manner. Unlike formal games, such as chess and Monopoly, games designed for educational purposes emphasize the process of play more than the outcome.

Problem-solving exercises, board games, and computer-assisted games are formats that have been used in simulation games. Problem-solving exercises provide a framework for solving a particular type of problem, generally by posing that specific problem and specifying a sequence of steps for solving it. For example, formulating a goal, assigning priorities, allocating resources and then distributing them might be a useful sequence. In board games, ideas or processes are represented by means of concrete symbols such as chips, markers and a game board. Learners investigate the processes by manipulating the symbols. In computer-assisted games the computer is used to calculate, store, and retrieve information, and to feed back mathematical or non-mathematical computation concerning players' judgments and decisions. By their nature, simulation games involve elements of both role playing and discussion. An important difference among the three lies in the degree of structure. Usually discussion is least structured. In role playing, some implicit behavior patterns are to be followed. In simulation games, explicit rules, similar to the regulations and procedures in an actual on-the-job setting, are to be followed.

There are several reasons one may decide to use simulation games in training. They offer an opportunity to learn by doing. The trainer teaches about selected aspects of life by having learners engage in them through a game. When games are done well, trainees become highly motivated and involved. Immediate feedback is available. Once the game rules are established, trainees can proceed without further assistance. Games encourage the student to learn because learning is directly pertinent to attaining goals.

One of the basic limitations of simulation games is that game play can involve considerable time. In addition, preparation of the game (that is, establishing the rules of play and developing the necessary supportive materials) usually requires considerable effort on the part of the instructor. One can, however, use a commercially available game.

Effective games have a number of characteristics. A successful game incorporates a fairly high degree of conflict and challenge. Often this is reflected by using limited resources to achieve strategic outcomes. An ideal simulation game imposes the fewest constraints on the player's behavior. Complicated and long rules are seldom appreciated by players. Effective games end well. It should be possible for all players to win, sometimes accomplished by having criteria for measuring success. The game should be realistic enough to involve the players. The situation should correspond to real life.

An effective simulation game should be replayable any number of times. This permits the players to try alternate strategies. A fast-paced simulation game can be very exciting. A majority of players prefer games of about 45 minutes. The game should be simple enough to learn quickly but complex enough to provide interest. Games that involve groups of three to five players are often more effective than those involving larger groups. An ideal game should involve aspects of motivation, instruction, evaluation and experimentation in proper balance. If instruction, simulation or gaming is emphasized out of proportion, the result may be a confusing, meaningless activity (Thiagerajan & Stolovitch, 1978). When contemplating the use of a simulation game, the first decision is whether the amount and kind of educational material to be covered will justify the effort required to construct the game. Once the decision has been made to proceed, select a format and then allow imagination full sway.

Sample Simulation Game

For purposes of illustration, a game for teaching the material used in the case study and role play examples can be used. One approach could be to create a deck of cards, each of which has a statement or two on it. Some statements would be appropriate to the occasion, and others would be either irrelevant or contraindicated. On the bottom of each card there would be a code referring to the scoring process. Players are each given five cards and each must draw a card from the rest of the deck each time it is his turn. A player must then choose a card to discard. After a predetermined number of rounds, participants are given a code and asked to add up their score. High score wins. The scoring code might work in the following fashion:

1. Cards with appropriate statements have the letter "A" followed by a number. The number refers to the points received, based on importance.
2. Cards with irrelevant statements have the letter "I" followed by dummy numbers. This means they will not be used in the scoring but must look no different from other cards.
3. Contraindicated statement cards will have the letter "C" followed by a number reflecting the degree of inappropriateness.

Players are told to total all "A" cards, then total all "C" cards, and disregard all "I" cards. They must subtract the "C" total from the "A" total. High score wins.

Simulation games can also be purchased. Several gerontology centers have developed games concerning retirement, service delivery, and other aspects of growing old.

Summary

Case study, role play, and simulation games can be effective alternatives to the more common lecture, demonstration, and discussion methods. They have a high degree of participant involvement and can be used for a variety of topics. They are particularly effective for training that involves feelings and attitudes in that they allow the participants to actively feel what a given situation is like. They are alternatives that can produce meaningful and interesting training.

Chapter 7
Outside Resources

Fortunately, the inservice coordinator will find most communities a rich source of resources. There are many agencies with intact programs that can be presented to the nursing home staff. Others will be happy to develop an inservice specific to the needs of nursing home personnel. Some of the resources you may wish to explore in your community are:

- Community college courses
- Outside lecture consultants
- Training corporations
- Commercial companies (i.e., drug companies)
- Trainers from other nursing homes with special expertise
- Health department consultation
- Physicians
- Clergy
- Pharmacists
- Fire department

- Red Cross (has lists of other community resources)
- Commission for the Blind (talking books are often available)
- Commission for the Deaf
- Visually impaired veterans
- Dentist and local dental societies
- Local library
- Local programs for the disabled
- Professional organizations (e.g., physical/occupational therapists)

At the same time, people within your facility can be used as trainers. Some of these resource people are:

- LVN
- RN
- Director of nurses
- Physical therapist
- Head of housekeeping (staff)
- Maintenance manager (staff)
- Dietary staff
- Activities director
- Business office staff
- Administrator
- Assistant administrator
- Trainees

An aide who has recently successfully completed a course can be asked to help another aide who may be just starting. Simple demonstrations, such as bed making or temperature recording, can be taught in this manner. This technique also gives the inservice director an additional way of checking on previous training. One of the best ways to reinforce training is to ask a trainee to explain the procedure to someone else.

Resource people, either within or outside your facility, can prove to be an invaluable help to health care professionals;

often they provide a new point of view, bring up-to-date information to the trainees, and generally lend variety to the training program.

Less often volunteers are used for training sessions. When nursing homes are able to develop a good volunteer program, many different forms of service should be available. There may be volunteers who have had experience in the classroom and would welcome an opportunity to help. Some training sessions may be recorded, others may be self-instructional. A volunteer may be able to conduct these types of inservice. Portions of the orientation, such as a guided tour of the facility, may be handled by volunteers. As already stated, resource people are abundant when you begin to comb the community.

No matter what resource is chosen, whether the person is inside or outside the facility, there are some guidelines to follow:

1. The trainer should select the areas in which it seems most desirable to involve an outside speaker, and should then choose possible resource people.
2. The trainer should contact the resource people and provide the following information: number and level of learners; time allowed for inservice; and objectives and expected outcomes. The trainer should provide information on anything else the resource person may need to know for planning.
3. The fee for the resource person, if any, should be agreed upon. It is usually courteous to reimburse travel expenses if there is not a consultant fee or if the resource person is part of a volunteer organization.
4. The trainer should draw up a written list of tentative objectives for the inservice and give them to the resource person.
5. The resource person should give the trainer an outline of the proposed inservice and a list of materials or equipment that will be needed.
6. The trainer should respond in writing to the resource per-

son. The letter should include objectives, outline, participants, time, date, and fee. Any evaluation or other planned activities should also be mentioned.
7. The trainer is responsible for identifying learners and for ensuring that they arrive on time and are prepared to participate.
8. After the training session, the trainer should summarize the information and translate it for use within the facility.

The use of outside resource people in staff development is a common approach to enhancing inservice programs. Outside resources can provide a means to bring experience and expertise to bear on immediate needs. They can share experiences from other facilities and bring a new depth and interest to a training program. The mere stimulus of a new face, a new voice, or a new approach can provide the motivation and excitement needed to make a training program more effective. Typically, an outside resource presents a prepared program using lecture and demonstration methods. Sometimes simulations or case studies will be included. Often the program has been designed and presented previously at other locations. Two specific ways in which resource persons may be utilized deserve some discussion. One method is the guest interview, and the other is a panel presentation.

Interview

The interview is an alternative to the guest lecture. The interview may be a better technique in a particular instance if the guest is not a good lecturer, or if he is likely to cover points already covered. The interview is, ideally, an informal, conversational technique. During the interview the audience listens as an interviewer asks a resource person specific questions about a prearranged topic. The interview is conversational in tone, in that the interviewer is free to improvise questions as the topic is explored.

The resource person is informed of the nature of the questions beforehand through a list of proposed review questions. An actual rehearsal of the interview is not necessary.

An interview is most appropriate for programs in which the objective is to clarify confusing issues and to present the impressions of an authority. Trainers concerned with providing a relaxed atmosphere for learning and stimulating interest should consider this technique.

The advantages of an interview are multiple. Resource persons may prefer the interview technique to the lecture. The interviewer is free to ask the resource person to clarify or give examples as the interview progresses. The interviewer maintains control of the subject matter discussed. The interview is not difficult to arrange, and it is often more interesting to listen to than is the lecture. The interview ensures continuity in the inservice programs and provides for audience participation if the trainer asks for questions from the listeners.

There are some limitations to consider. Certain topics do not lend themselves to an interview. Detailed information is difficult to present and comprehend. Some people cannot adjust to the interview approach. The resource person may lapse into giving speeches instead of short and direct answers. The audience may feel left out if they are not involved when preparing questions.

In arranging the interview, an interviewer's first priority is to determine the objectives for the inservice program and to make certain that the interview technique is appropriate to the topic and objectives. Once decided, the search for an appropriate resource person in the community or, if needed, outside the community should be undertaken. Well in advance of the interview, the interviewer should, with the help of the staff, prepare a list of possible questions to be discussed.

When the trainer contacts the resource person, the two

should review the questions and come to an understanding of the range of the subject matter to be discussed and the purposes of the interview. The resource person has the privilege of eliminating questions or adding some that will help to clarify the issue. The interviewer should make certain that the resource person is aware of the audience's background and knowledge of the topic, as well as of the procedure that will be followed in asking and responding to questions.

The interviewer should also arrange for the room, sound system and other equipment, and should make certain that the audience will have comfortable seating. Finally, the trainer or interviewer should prepare an introduction for the interview, in which topic and length of the interview, and the background and qualifications of the resource person are explained.

The interviewer allows the speaker to feel comfortable and to warm up to the topic by spending a few minutes of general introduction. The interviewer should ask clear, concise questions and should clarify remarks; the resource person should answer as clearly as possible, using a vocabulary suited to the audience. Speeches and pet theories should be avoided unless they are appropriate to the interview.

If a question and answer period is to follow, the audience may want to take a few notes during the interview or jot down questions they would like to have addressed.

Sample Interview

The administration plans to purchase new equipment for taking temperature and blood pressure, and the decision is made to buy electric skin thermometers and automated electronic sphygmomanometers. The nursing staff may have questions about the efficacy of adopting the new technology. Therefore, an interview with the director of nurses from another facility where this equipment is already in use is arranged. In order to accomplish this, the inservice director would:

1. Gather information on the concerns of the staff, including any specific questions they may have.
2. Consolidate this information, along with what is at issue from a teaching point of view, into a list of questions.
3. Contact the director of nurses at the other facility and review the questions and concerns.
4. Make any arrangements needed for visual aides that the visiting director of nurses may need, including actual equipment.
5. Prepare the introduction, explaining that the proposed new equipment will be discussed by someone who is familiar with its use.

The final interview might include this type of interchange:

Interviewer: We are wondering if this new equipment won't be more difficult to use?

Director: We found this to be true in a few cases, until aides became familiar with it. However, at present we feel there is a time savings as the result of using the newer methods.

Interviewer: I'm wondering how difficult it will be to retrain everyone in a different method?

Director: We were surprised to find that one inservice was all that was needed for the majority, and a second review session took care of any who still felt unsure.

Interviewer: The electric skin thermometer is so much more cumbersome than a glass thermometer; we have some concern it will make the aide's job more difficult.

Director: Actually, our aides report there is less work involved than the vigorous shaking required by the glass thermometer. I've brought one with me, and I will be happy to pass it around so you can see how lightweight it is. Notice it is battery operated, and therefore you have no electric cord to worry about.

At any point questions from the group can be answered. Otherwise, the interview would continue until the prepared questions had been answered.

Panel Discussion

The panel, another alternative to the guest lecture, is a small group of persons who discuss a topic with the guidance of a moderator. The moderator prepares questions to begin the discussion and to keep it going. The audience does not verbally participate unless specifically requested to do so. The panel can best be used to bring several points of view into focus for the audience, and it is an especially good technique for clarifying controversial issues. Because participants are chosen for their expertise in a given field, the panel makes optimum use of a wide range of opinion.

The moderator guides the discussion through a series of questions and comments. Obviously the moderator should be familiar with the topic discussed. The panel members are selected to represent different backgrounds and a variety of points of view and should be good conversationalists. Care should be taken to avoid debates while on the panel. Members are chosen because of their ability to speak with some authority on the subject, either because of past or present experiences.

Advantages of panels are that several informed opinions can be heard rather than just one, and several competent resource persons can participate. Audience interest is stimulated through the discussion technique. The limitations to panels are that panel members who are familiar with the topic may be hard to find, and an uninformed or unskilled moderator may have difficulty keeping the discussion going.

In arranging the panel discussion, the moderator of the panel must determine the goals of the discussion well in advance. Once the objectives are decided, the trainer or moderator should understand both the topic to be discussed and the points of view of the audience members. The moderator prepares an introduction in which panel members are briefly introduced, and prepares questions to open and sustain the discussion. A meeting with panel members beforehand to be sure they understand the panel procedure and the range of the topic to be discussed is desirable. A review of the names of panel members, the goals of the panel, time restrictions, and seating locations is also needed.

During the panel discussion the moderator's responsibility is to keep the conversation flowing among the participants. After giving a prepared introduction, the moderator guides the informal discussion through questions and comments and offers a chance for all members to participate. The moderator remains neutral, summarizes points, and reminds panel members of any time limits. Panel members gear their discussion to the audience and avoid lengthy, involved answers that dominate the time.

If a question and answer period is to follow, the audience may want to take a few notes during the panel or write down questions they would like to have addressed. Participants and audience members should be comfortably seated, and extremes in room temperature should be avoided.

Sample Panel

Consider the possibility that differing opinions were found when other professionals were approached on the use of the proposed new equipment (using the same example as used in the sample above). In this case, arranging an informal panel composed of people who have had experience with electric skin temperature machines and electronic blood pressure machines, but with different advice to give regarding their acquisition, is desirable. The procedure would be as follows:

1. Select the panel members to represent the respective views involved.
2. Prepare an introduction and questions to open and sustain the discussion. These should cover the main points in controversy such as ease of use, time consumed, patient response, upkeep, and accuracy.
3. Advise the members of the procedure for conducting the panel. Include the topics that will be covered in the introduction and sustaining types of questions. Make sure panel members understand the time limitations.
4. Questions from the group and a general acknowledgment that the subject was covered adequately can be an effective summary.

Summary

There are many ways to utilize outside resources. They vary from standard training already developed by companies and agencies to a highly inventive use of volunteers. Variety in training can be the result of using outside resources. Most trainers find outside resource people stimulating. As training director you may also find you are continuing to learn from the resource people. Also, utilizing the community enhances the relationship between it and the nursing home.

Chapter 8
Review and Practice

Once new material has been presented and learning has begun, the techniques of review and practice become increasingly important to trainers. Although practice and review are time-tested techniques of teaching and are essential to every subject area, they are easily misused and can, therefore, be ineffective.

The purpose of the review or practice is to help learners apply original concepts to related job situations. If trainers neglect this relationship between original learning and its application to real life, the review or practice sessions will be directionless.

Review

A review is exactly what the word implies—a re-view, or re-look, at information already presented through some teaching method (for example, lecture, discussion, demonstration).

Ideally, reviews give learners an opportunity to find new meanings and new ways of understanding already learned concepts by helping learners to transfer those concepts to real-life situations.

Most reviews are appropriate at the end of a unit of content. Basic concepts from the unit are brought together in a logical order, clarified, and expanded to apply to related situations. An appropriate review should generate considerable enthusiasm and creativity in the learners who, once they understand how the concepts they have studied can be applied to job situations, become more interested in learning.

Planning is essential to prevent poor review sessions. Trainers should go to great lengths to plan reviews so that original concepts are extended to on-the-job situations. Examples from learners, personal experiences, simulations, and other methods can be used as illustrations.

There are a number of advantages to use of the review as a teaching method. Review eases the application or transfer of learning to related situations and, thus, the learning can become more permanent. Misconceptions and misunderstandings can be corrected during the review phase. Basically, review is a flexible procedure that can last as little as a few minutes or for as long as several class sessions. The important point is that review provides feedback and reinforcement and thus aids learning.

Review, however, can be misused. Too often, recitation is substituted for review. If learners have not developed a good understanding of the material, review is pointless. But review can evaluate whether or not learners understand content. Last, if a test follows a review, the test must contain questions that evaluate application of concepts to on-the-job situations, not recall of isolated facts.

The review can be used for something as global as the overall policies of the institution or something as specific as a routine for handling unexpected problems.

Practice

The importance of practice or drill for developing particular skills cannot be overemphasized. Every skill demands practice, whether it be as elementary as delivering meal trays or as complicated as changing dressings. A person who does not practice a newly learned skill may be able to repeat the skill, but he will never reach full capacity for performance.

Educators have found that skills are best developed through the three steps of initial learning, varied content, and repetitive practice. In initial learning the purpose of the skill is explained and verbal instructions are given. Often a demonstration is included. The next step is direct contact with the skill through a variety of situations. During this phase learners develop and test their own ways of performing the skill. The trainer helps to minimize weaknesses and to perfect strengths. Through repetitive practice, which varies conditions under which a skill is repeated to avoid monotony and increase the likelihood of its transfer to related situations, the skill is perfected. Practice is the basic instructional method for getting and developing mental and motor skills. It allows trainers to practice with learners one at a time and when spaced appropriately, practice can help reduce the rate of forgetting. Practice develops habits that tend to become part of one. Practice, however, is not effective for certain kinds of learning, and misguided practice may actually hinder learning. Striking a balance between speed and accuracy is difficult. Repetitive drill may become monotonous. Working out practice sessions with each learner can sometimes be complicated and time consuming. Practice can be used effectively whether the behavior is one that is seldom necessary, such as evacuation, often necessary, such as transferring hemiplegic patients, or regularly necessary, such as bed making.

The techniques of review and practice are alike in that they both supplement concepts originally learned in the classroom. Both ensure more permanent learning. The two techniques are not equally appropriate for each situation, however. Reviews work best when the trainer is teaching cognitive or mental concepts; practice is appropriate when teaching particular behaviors or skills. Reviews involve the whole class; practice must be one-to-one for best results. Reviews can be used when teaching such things as the policies of the facility, department, or unit; characteristics of geriatric patients; or the steps in reporting an incident. Practice can be used for such things as the procedures involved in an evacuation plan; transfer of hemiplegic patients; or taking vital signs.

Retention and Transfer

At this point, it may be important to examine some of the major aspects of retention and transfer for incorporation into instructional methods. Kenneth Hoover (1980, pp. 154-155) has described eleven major points:

1. The initial learning experiences are usually best retained. This means that as part of the instructional process, one should check for accuracy of initial reactions. It is difficult to correct the inaccurate reactions but it is better to correct them early in the instruction.
2. It is easiest to recall the original learning sequence whether one has learned mental or motor skills. By varying the sequencing and combinations, one can increase learning.
3. Forgetting occurs by degree. Approximately one third of material studied is retained for one year. The rate of forgetting is always greater immediately after learning. Despite forgetting, relearning is easily achieved.
4. The recall of specific facts is more difficult than the recall of the existence of the fact or the attitude or method associated with them.

5. Overlearning or learning beyond mastery increases retention. The amount of overlearning generally recommended is 50 percent. Additional practice exercises are often beneficial.
6. Recall after a brief rest is improved if learning is interrupted or stopped just prior to mastery. To enhance learning, do not fill the rest of the time with new material after the initial learning sequence is completed. It might be better to include more practice.
7. One lengthy practice session is not as beneficial as smaller sessions of varying length. Practice sessions of decreasing length with the rest periods in between seem to be most beneficial.
8. Transfer is enhanced when the trainer makes a conscious effort to teach for transfer.
9. Transfer of concepts, methods, and attitudes is achieved more easily than transfer of facts. Facts are transferred to new situations only if the new situations contain the same facts.
10. One learning experience may interfere with another. This can occur if there is similarity between the two situations. This is called negative transfer.
11. Negative transfer can be decreased when the corresponding elements are separated in both time and situation. Negative transfer can be minimized by increasing the thoroughness of learning and providing for overlearning.

Consideration of these principles can lead to more effective teaching and learning.

The importance of this element of training cannot be overemphasized. Many trainers become frustrated when they discover what they have taught is not being practiced once trainees are back on the job. Often this problem can be alleviated by sufficient review and/or practice. As Hoover (1980) points out, learning which occurs first in time (for example, at another facility) may be retained better than current instruction. Added to this is the tendency for the greatest amount of forgetting to occur immediately after the learning. During review and/or practice sessions, it may even be advantageous to coach trainees on how they can remember new procedures, how they can avoid the tendency to lapse into old ways, and so on. Overlearning can go a long way toward resolving ambivalent responses.

Chapter 9
Evaluation

Evaluation is the point at which the trainer determines whether or not the inservice program has met the goals of the nursing home. Because evaluation provides concrete feedback about what inservice has accomplished, it can provide the inservice trainer with information on ways in which programs should be changed to better meet the goals of the facility. If better patient care is the ultimate goal of inservice then the evaluation should focus on employee performance. An evaluation is the process of determining the learners' achievement of training objectives as well as the effectiveness and efficiency of the delivery system. The evaluation process should assess both the learners' competence and the program's efficacy.

The first step in conducting an evaluation is to determine the objectives of the program. Since written learner objectives have already been set forth during program planning, these same objectives can now be used to determine whether or not learners have achieved the desired level of performance.

Learners' progress should be measured throughout training, not just as the end of a program or series. Learners need to know their strengths and weaknesses. Deficiencies should be immediately corrected and not allowed to become habits. The trainer can advise and guide learners toward self-improvement if evaluation is done periodically.

Similarly, self-evaluation is important to the planner. An inservice director should want to know how well a program is serving its objectives as it goes along. This is called formative evaluation, and it takes place during development and try-outs. It is useful for determining any weaknesses in the plan that can be improved before full-scale use. Reactions from employees and supervisors, observations of trainees at work, and suggestions from colleagues may indicate deficiencies in such things as the learning sequence, procedures, materials, and so on. For example, the pace of instruction may be too slow; the sequence may be uninteresting, confusing, or too difficult. Formative evaluation also allows the supervisor to determine whether at any point in the instructional sequence too much previous knowledge has been assumed, or whether the emphasis is on material already mastered and not requiring more attention.

The careful analysis of the results of a program in full use is called a summative evaluation. It is concerned with evaluating the degree of final achievement of objectives. This is usually done through a post-test. It may also entail following up after a course is completed to determine if and how employees are using or applying the knowledge, skills, and attitudes treated in the program.

At this point in the evaluation, administration may be interested in accountability, or the effectiveness and efficiency of the inservice program. Feedback from summative evaluation should be used for revising and improving any parts of the instructional plan that need it. Evaluation can also provide data on the cost and benefits of inservice.

Measurement Techniques

Evaluation is not measurement. The trainer must elect an appropriate measurement technique for providing the information upon which inservice program decisions will be based. A number of measurement techniques were presented in Chapter 3. Questionnaires, interviews, job analysis, reports, tests, and group problem techniques can all be used as measures for evaluation. However, the measurement technique most appropriate for inservice is the performance test. Performance tests assess learners' ability to demonstrate competency in performing skills, tasks, and procedures. Performance tests should correspond to the learning objectives. The checklist, records, and simulation are three other types of performance tests that are easy to use in the nursing home setting.

Checklist

A checklist is a prepared list of statements related to particular attitudes, actions, or performance standards. Checklists can be completed by the learner, a supervisor, or by the trainer. The responses can be in formats such as "yes/no," "acceptable/ unacceptable," or "satisfactory/needs improvement/unsatisfactory."

Records

Records can be regularly reviewed by the trainer. Written logs of training should be kept. These provide the trainer with a record of what worked or did not work, any problems which occurred, good questions, and areas needing more review. Floor records, incidents, complaints, and employee files are also records that can be used for evaluation.

Simulation

Simulation is a performance assessment that enables the learner to demonstrate a particular skill in a realistic setting. Simulations allow learners to test skills and judgments in the context of reality; to get prompt and specific feedback on performance without risk to patients; to try several approaches; to practice; and to work on one part of a complex problem at a time. Basically, simulation allows the learner to participate and practice a technique until it is perfected.

Sample Evaluation

Directions: Please rate each of your aides on the following tasks.

Task	Performs well				Performs poorly
	1	2	3	4	5
1. Choose correct type of thermometer (rectal/oral)	___	___	___	___	___
2. Observe proper care of thermometer	___	___	___	___	___
3. Take an oral temperature using correct procedures	___	___	___	___	___
4. Take a rectal temperature using correct procedures	___	___	___	___	___
5. Record temperature correctly	___	___	___	___	___

The nurse on a particular wing was asked to rate each of the twelve aides on that wing on the above tasks. It was determined through the needs analysis (see Chapter 3) that review and practice were needed for Task 4 and a re-training session was needed for Task 5. The learning objectives corresponding to these tasks were:

- Each aide will be able to demonstrate the correct method of taking a rectal temperature.
- Each aide will be able to correctly record the temperature reading from ten written examples of thermometers.

For purposes of review, practice, and retraining, the trainer can then provide an inservice which includes these two objectives. At the end of the training, each aide is asked to complete the following checklist.

Directions: Please rate each of your aides on the following tasks.

Task	Can do well	Need more training	Cannot do well
	1	2	3
1. Choose correct type of thermometer (rectal/oral)	___	___	___
2. Observe proper care of thermometer	___	___	___
3. Take an oral temperature using correct procedures	___	___	___
4. Take a rectal temperature using correct procedures	___	___	___
5. Record temperature correctly	___	___	___

The nurse then rates the aides again. If both the nurse and the aides feel that performance on these tasks is now acceptable, the training can be evaluated as successful. This is an example of the way in which a checklist can be used in evaluating training.

Several other things should be considered by the inservice trainer during evaluation. Objectives should be evaluated: Are the objectives really matched to learner needs? Method of presentation should be evaluated: Is the method of presentation appropriate? And inservice goals should be evaluated: Is inservice meeting the goals of the nursing home?

Trainers should be particularly careful not to attempt to measure learner reactions to presentation techniques as an evaluation of overall training. This is bound for failure. Unless the popularity of a particular presentation is being measured, trainee performance alone must be the criterion.

Summary

In summary, the following three points should be considered in evaluation:

1. the degree to which training prepared learners to perform particular job functions (learner evaluation);
2. the degree to which the objectives were achieved (program evaluation);
3. information concerning learner feedback on method of presentation (diagnostic tool).

This leads to one of the three following evaluation decisions:

1. Continue inservice as is; no problems.
2. Discontinue current inservice; too many problems.
3. Modify, revise, and expand current inservice; some things are working well, others are not, and new problems have been identified.

Chapter 10
Inservice Benefits
to the Nursing Home

Inservice education is the major mechanism by which the administrator communicates the nursing home's philosophy, policies, and procedures. New employees can be oriented to the values and priorities which stem from an identified philosophy of care. The overall goals that all employees will be expected to work toward are usually explained in the orientation training. The translation of these goals into patient care policy, personnel policy, and public relations (including family relations) policy is also conveyed during training. The way in which the nursing home's policies are to be effected is the bulk of the content of inservice instruction either on the job or in the classroom. In this way the administrative foundation is integrated into the functioning of the facility. Therefore, successful administrators are quite aware of the potential benefits of inservice education for coordinating and integrating philosophy, policy and resident care.

Practical matters such as employee dissatisfaction and

disloyalty are everyday concerns of the nursing home administrator. Disgruntled or disengaged employees are often those who contribute to the costly turnover rate. At best, they may conduct subtle sabotage operations such as a waste of supplies, "accidental" spillage and breakage and, too frequently, petty theft. Here, too, inservice education can be beneficial. Many dissatisfactions stem from inadequate employee orientation and training. As a result, employees are not fully integrated into the facility, and they know it. It then becomes entirely too easy to take advantage of the nursing home administration.

In the nursing home setting, the staff who deliver hands-on care is very often made up of hourly wage earners. These employees often have little background or experience working in nursing homes. Even if they have worked previously in nursing homes, the difference in policies and procedures from one home to another can be confusing. This type of employee is many times hired in response to staffing needs demanded by regulations. The orientation provided them is far too brief, yet performance expectations are high and are not altered by the difficult circumstances arising from continual turnover. Employees handled in this manner do not perceive themselves as really belonging to the staff or as being closely affiliated with the institution; thus, turnover rates remain high.

Furthermore, staff on all levels are prone to be uneducated in the field of aging and chronic illness. Thus, they often do not know how to handle problems which they encounter. This can lead to defensive behaviors usually resulting in poor patient care. It is also a source of low morale among the employees caused by constant job frustration.

For all the reasons above it is imperative that thorough orientation and on-the-job training be offered to these employees. Inservice offers a continuing opportunity for staff to develop competencies and become aware of the interdisciplinary nature of patient care. Since the needs of older patients are multiple, it is necessary to develop care plans which reflect the knowledge of multiple care givers interacting on the patients' behalf. This maximizes patient care while giving employees the satisfaction of knowing that their individual contributions are necessary to the total plan. Each care giver's effort may appear minimal in view of the complexity and severity of needs a given resident may have; however, when viewed as part of an interacting total plan of care, all facets of care giving are seen as important to the goals.

Most directors of nurses find themselves spending a considerable amount of time counseling single employees concerning job performance and expectations. Surveys show that this aspect of the director of nurses' job is least liked and is seen as interfering most with nursing duties. Therefore, job satisfaction decreases for both the director of nurses and other employees. Successful orientation and inservice can alleviate the waste of professional time, with better employee morale as the result.

With these thoughts in mind, what can the inservice trainer do within his nursing home to ensure that inservice will benefit the facility and increase the quality of patient care? First of all, effective training must transfer from the classroom to the job. This means that there must be a close connection between the two. Adult training needs support to survive; otherwise it is doomed to failure. An adult learner is someone who has already overlearned certain behaviors. All adult training is an unequal competition with preexisting habits, especially those habits which are supported by simply conforming to whatever one's peers are doing and to what one's supervisors expect or condone.

Pretraining support is essential. Minor behavior changes are more likely to be accomplished than are major changes. Training that attempts to extend existing habits or implant ideas consistent with those already known and understood is more likely to work than is training that tries to replace an old repertoire of habits with an entire new repertoire. Training, therefore, should not be overly ambitious. One small step at a time is more beneficial than no steps or steps backward.

Training should be useful. The trainer should carefully analyze learner needs to discover what behaviors already exist and how to make use of preexisting behaviors within training. The reasons for training must be readily apparent to trainees. In one sense, training is an intrusion into existing behavior. Therefore, trainees need to understand and support the reasons for training. This is no problem when the trainee is a beginner who has no skills, but it can be a serious problem for retraining or for training employees who are moving from one nursing home to another.

Planning for training includes tailoring the programs to meet the specific behaviors and understood needs of the group. Then training is more likely to be accepted, and the behaviors practiced during the training program have a better chance of transferring to the job.

The trainer can also impact the learners. Often a learner will remember more about an instructor than about content. Behaviors modeled by the trainer can have a powerful impact on the learner. Instructor behavior that does not reinforce the instructional content produces feelings of discomfort within a learner. This can result in the learner discounting the importance and job relevancy of the content.

Following are the five trainer behaviors that increase motivation to learn:

1.   Maintain and enhance the self-esteem of the learners.
2.   Focus on learners' behaviors and not on learners' personalities.
3.   Actively listen.
4.   Use positive reinforcement to shape learning.
5.   Set goals and follow-up dates and maintain communications (Rosenbaum & Baker, 1979).

No training supports itself and unsupported learning inevitably dies. Old learning is supported by force of habit. At best, all that classroom training accomplishes is to prepare the learner to benefit from on-the-job feedback and reinforcement.

A trainer must ensure that feedback and reinforcement be incorporated in training. Appeals for support should be directed to those persons within the facility who must act differently if training is to have an impact. The appeal should be based on the ability of the learners to do their jobs better. One example of this is supervisor support. Instead of approaching the facility's administrator, the trainer should approach the LVNs, explain what will be included in the next inservice for aides, and give a quick demonstration. Suggestions and feedback should be asked for, and training modified whenever it is appropriate. Then all LVNs should be encouraged to watch for and reward the expected new behavior with a positive comment.

The people whose behavior has the greatest impact on trainees' behavior are those with the most frequent daily contact. A new employee should be assigned a well-trained "buddy" to support correct patient care procedures. Reinforcement and reward need not be extensive or expensive. On the contrary, it is usually sufficient simply to acknowledge that someone is doing what is expected.

Work with the administration to establish some job incentives will ensure that the reinforcement will be more than a simple positive statement. A visible interest in staff development can help. The building of a certain sense of camaraderie is beneficial. Practically speaking, in the nursing home setting, one must often find ways of persuading people to do well the work that they would rather not do at all. It is helpful to periodically remind people of the reasons that the job has to be done in a certain manner, of ways that they as individuals fit within the structure of overall patient care, and of their importance to the facility and the patients. Explanations will, however, not make the work more attractive. Training cannot make the work more pleasant, but it can make the work easier to perform and less oppressive. Explanations, praise, and support of and from all levels of employees can make an overall impact on positive patient care.

Another important aspect of inservice education involves the development of the staff. A good program will offer opportunities for employees to develop greater expertise. Review and practice allows employees to develop proficiency on the job. Teaching new methods and sharing new knowledge allows them to keep up to date. Encouraging well-trained employees to help with the training affords them an opportunity to develop new skills. Often inservice programs include leadership training. For some employees this will be the needed impetus for career advancement. These factors all work together to provide a more qualified staff. The result is better care. Eventually, good care attracts more residents, and an increased revenue can enable the administrator to improve workers' benefits.

Inservice education can be utilized to meet employees' higher order needs. In particular, discussions and feedback which occur during training can give employees a sense of belonging to the organization. Employees can enjoy a feeling of self-worth when their suggestions are heeded and their input utilized. As Maslow (1970) has pointed out, the meeting of those higher order needs permits individuals to feel self-fulfilled. Staff members who obtain this type of satisfaction on the job are not only likely to remain with the facility, but will also tend toward better job performance.

Finally, good inservice education can be an excellent public relations vehicle. Well-informed, dedicated employees are one vital link to the community. They will communicate what is really happening at the nursing home, and they will educate the general public. The better informed the staff, the better the impression in the community. Unfortunately, there is a widespread negative stereotype about nursing homes. Employees who have been well trained and enjoy working in nursing homes can do much to dispel the popular myths surrounding them.

In conclusion, the benefits of inservice for the staff are (United Hospital Fund of New York, 1972):

1. promoting understanding and commitment to the goals of the home, through orientation programming;
2. providing satisfactions by developing the skills needed to do a good job on a continuing basis;
3. offering the additional satisfaction of the human desire for growth and development by providing refresher information and training in new skills;
4. giving staff a chance to grow with their jobs and to take on additional responsibilities by offering courses in leadership and management development;
5. actively involving staff members in checking on their own levels of performance and in setting higher standards of on-the-job performance;
6. promoting mutual respect for each other's work roles and responsibilities by giving personnel from various disciplines opportunities to exchange ideas and information and to solve problems together.

The benefits for the nursing home include the following:

1. Inservice education can promote a higher level of patient/resident care and can develop a more efficient and loyal staff.
2. It can improve the public image of the home, and of nursing homes in general, within the immediate community.
3. It can also provide a new perception of the nursing home as a laboratory for analyzing problems and working out

practical solutions to the problems of delivering care and services to chronically ill and aging residents.
4. It can also develop a neutral environment in which interpersonal and interdepartmental disagreements can be resolved, and where staff turnover can be reduced.

Inservice education is instrumental in developing human resources needed to provide care and services that satisfy the complex needs of personnel, residents, families, and the community. Inservice education is a continuing responsibility shared by administrative and other personnel responsible for the safety and well-being of nursing home residents and staff.

References

Allen, D.W. and Seifman, E. *The teacher's handbook.* Glenview, Ill.: Scott, Foresman & Company, 1971.

American Hospital Association. *Media handbook: A guide to selecting, producing, and using media for patient educacation programs.* Chicago: American Hospital Association, 1978.

Cooper, J.M., et al. *Classroom teaching skills: A handbook.* Lexington, Me.: D.C. Heath and Company, 1977.

Dale, Edgar. *Audio-visual methods in teaching, rev. ed.* New York: Dryden, 1954.

Freedman, C.R. *Teaching patients.* San Diego, Ca.: Courseware, Inc., 1978.

Gunning, R. *The technique of clear writing,* rev. ed., New York: McGraw-Hill, 1968.

Hoover, K.H. *College teaching today: A handbook for post-secondary instruction.* Boston: Allyn and Bacon, Inc., 1980.

Knowles, M. *The Modern practice of adult education: Andragogy versus pedagogy.* New York: Association Press, 1970.

Mager, Robert F. *Preparing instructional objectives,* 2nd edition. Palo Alto, Ca.: Fearon-Pitman Publishers, Inc., 1975.

Maslow, A.H. *Motivation and personality*, 2nd edition. New York: Harper & Row, 1970.

Rogers, C. *Freedom to learn: A view of what education might be*. Columbus, Oh.: C.E. Merrill Publishing Co., 1969.

Rosenbaum, B.L., and Baker, B. Do as I do: The trainer as a behavior model. *Training/HRD* (Dec. 1979), pp. 89-93.

Thiagerajan, S. and Stolovitch, H. *Instructional simulation games*. Englewood Cliffs, NJ: Educational Technology Publications, 1978.

United Hospital Fund of New York. *A concept in inservice education in nursing homes*. New York: Nursing Home Trainer Program NYM/RMP Project #20 61-70 A, 1972.

Suggested Readings

The authors have found the following list of books helpful and informative in gathering the information for this book, in teaching staff development, and for use in teaching students to conduct nursing home staff development.

Cassella, C. *Training exercises to improve interpersonal relations in health care organizations.* New York: Panel Publishers, 1977.

Clark, C.C. *The nurse as continuing educator.* New York: Springer Publishing Company, 1979.

Clark, C.C. *The nurse as group leader.* New York: Springer Publishing Company, 1977.

Dick, W. and Carey, L. *The systematice design of instruction.* Glenview, Il.: Scott, Foresman and Company, 1978.

Donaldson, L. *Behavioral supervision: Practical ways to change unsatisfactory behavior and increase productivity.* Reading, Ma.: Addison-Wesley Publishing Company, 1980.

Foley, R.P. and Smilansky, J. *Teaching techniques: A handbook for health professionals.* New York: McGraw-Hill, 1980.

Fordyce, J.K. and Weil, R. *Managing with people*, 2nd ed. Reading, Ma.: Addison-Wesley, 1979.

Hoover, K. *College teaching today: A handbook for post-secondary instruction.* Boston: Allyn and Bacon, Inc., 1976.

Ingalls, J.D. *A trainer's guide to Andragogy*, Washington, D.C.: U.S. Department of Health, Education, and Welfare, HE 17.8: AN2/973, 1973.

Knowles, M. *The adult learner: A neglected species*, 2nd ed. Houston: Gulf Publishing Company, 1979.

Laird, D. *Approaches to training and development.* Reading, Ma.: Addison-Wesley Publishing Company, 1978.

Lemke, R., Standke, L. and Jones, P. *Designing and delivering cost-effective training—and measuring the results.* Minneapolis, Mn.: Lakewood publications, 1981.

Linton, C.B. and Truelove, J.W. *Hospital-based education.* New York: Arco Publishing Co., 1980.

Loughary, J.W. and Hopson, B. *Producing workshops, seminars, short courses: A trainer's handbook.* Chicago: Follett Publishing Company, 1979.

McKeachie, W. *Teaching tips: A guidebook for the beginning college teacher*, 7th ed. Lexington, Ma.: D.C. Heath and Company, 1978.

Media handbook: A guide to selecting, producing, and using media for patient education programs. Chicago: American Hospital Association, 1978.

Miller, H.G. and Verduia, J.R. *The adult educator.* Houston: Gulf Publishing Co., 1979.

Redman, B.K. *The process of patient teaching in nursing*, 4th ed. St. Louis: C.V. Mosby Co., 1980.

Sampson, E.E. and Marthas, M.S. *Group processes for the health professions.* New York: John Wiley and Sons, 1977.

Tobin, H.M., Yoder, P.S., Yoder Wise, P.S. and Hull, P.K. *The process of staff development: Components for change.* St. Louis: C.V. Mosby Co., 1979.

Trecker, H.B. and Trecker, A.R. *Working with groups, committees, and communities*. Chicago: Follett Publishing Co., 1979.

Weil, M. and Joyce, B. *Social models of teaching: Expanding your teaching repertoire*. Englewood Cliffs, NJ: Prentice-Hall, Inc., 1978.

Index